Safe Sex in the Garden

AND OTHER PROPOSITIONS
FOR AN ALLERGY-FREE WORLD

Thomas Leo Ogren

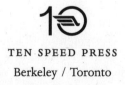

TEN SPEED PRESS
Berkeley / Toronto

Ten Speed Press
P.O. Box 7123
Berkeley, California 94707
www.tenspeed.com

Distributed in Australia by Simon and Schuster Australia, in Canada by Ten Speed Press Canada, in New Zealand by Southern Publishers Group, in South Africa by Real Books, and in the United Kingdom and Europe by Airlift Book Company.

Cover design by Jeff Clark, Wilsted & Taylor Publishing Services
Cover illustration by Berthe Hoola Van Nooten
Text design by Valerie Brewster

LIBRARY OF CONGRESS CATALOGING-IN-PUBLICATION DATA
Ogren, Thomas Leo.
  Safe sex in the garden: and other propositions for an allergy-free world / Thomas Leo Ogren.
   p. cm.
  ISBN 1-58008-314-5 (pbk.)
   1. Low-allergen gardens. 2. Low-allergen plants. 3. Plants, Sex in. 1. Title.
  SB433.4.O48 2003
  635.9 – DC21   2002156527

First printing, 2003
Printed in Canada

1 2 3 4 5 6 7 8 9 10 – 07 06 05 04 03

This book is dedicated to two of the most wonderful
and supportive people I have ever had the profound pleasure to know—
my grandmother, Norma Myers, and my good friend and mentor,
the playwright Ronald Alexander.

ACKNOWLEDGMENTS

I would like to thank some of the many people who helped me gather this information and write this book. Special thanks are due Walter and Memory Lewis, the remarkable husband-wife team of botanist and microbiologist who have been so supportive and quick to lend a hand. I have also been extremely lucky to have the wise counsel of retired allergist David A. Stadtner, M.D., a doctor who understands the role that plants so often play in allergies.

This book, like my last one, has been a true family affair. My parents, Bud and Paula Ogren, fine editors both, have been totally supportive, encouraging and always there when needed. My sister Liz contributed many innovative, important ideas, and her husband, Professor Dan Krieger, has also long been an incredible help.

My brothers David and Paul have likewise been solidly behind me. Paul, who understands plant flowering systems and their relationship to health better than anyone I know, continues to find and share new material that is completely invaluable.

My sister Rachel Clark has been helping me with this work for many years now, as has my youngest sister, budding botanist and artist Mary Rose Ogren-O'Leary. Special thanks to Sherryl Cantor Ogren, who came up with the title for this book. My children – Sarah, Hildur, Naomi, and Josh–have not only been supportive and helpful in the many years of research, but each of them has consistently made me proud with their discipline, drive, and hunger for education. Sarah and Hildur, our twins, are my literary agents for this book and are due special thanks for their buoyant optimism, their hands-on help with the proposal, and also for selling my last book.

I'd like to thank Kirsty Melville, the publisher at Ten Speed Press, for having the foresight to put this work in print. Everyone at Ten Speed Press has always been totally approachable, including the owner, Phil Wood. I feel very lucky to be associated with this progressive, high-quality press. Special thanks are due my editor for this book, Meghan Keeffe, for her creative advice and no-nonsense editing.

I want to thank the folks from the American Lung Association in Richmond, Virginia, who made their chapter the first to landscape with pollen-free plants.

Thanks too must go to dear friend and fellow author "Uppity Woman" Vicki Leon for her editing, advice, and concern. I would also like to thank garden writer and biologist Carol Deppe for her excellent contributions. As a teacher I've been blessed with a great many wonderful students over the years, but perhaps none has been smarter or more dedicated than Rachele Melious. For being available with help and valuable advice at all hours of the night on a multitude of computer problems, I wish to thank Lynda Cokeley.

And last (well, almost), a few people in particular have helped me to keep my sanity and sense of humor as I tried to pull this all together. My good friends Shelby Stover, Ray Oblouk, and Johnny Banks have always helped to keep things fun.

And then last but certainly not least, my wife, Yvonne, who has been my best friend all these years. Yvonne has kept me on track, has taken care of virtually all the thousands of things most other folks have to do, and has made it possible for me to roam far afield collecting pollen, plants, and photographs. Yvonne does almost everything for me, and this has freed me to research and write.

Many people told me that my research was so unusual and important that I'd soon be rich and famous. Well, I'm getting known, but I'm hardly famous, and as for rich, I already was. Not with money, mind you, but rich in family, in health, in friendship, in love; rich in being able to totally pursue something that deeply interests me. Truthfully, no one should wish for more.

CONTENTS

A man with a new idea is a crank
until the idea succeeds.
MARK TWAIN

A few months ago I was asked to come to some people's house to make recommendations as to the allergy potential of their landscape. I don't do too much of this personal consulting since I'm usually too busy with writing, research, or giving lectures, but this request was local, and the man had read my book, *Allergy-Free Gardening,* so I agreed. He was a computer programmer, and his wife was an English professor. The wife had occasional allergies, but the husband suffered greatly for much of the year. Their existing landscape had come with the house, and they were open to making any changes that I would suggest.

Every time I do an evaluation of a landscape I find that each yard is different, presenting different problems. I found several large male junipers growing in their rather weedy low-maintenance front yard. I suggested they get rid of the male junipers and replace them with female ones. I also suggested that they plant more plants so that there would be less bare ground – less room for weeds to grow. Additional mulch was also recommended.

When I am doing a consultation like this one, I am always hoping to find a smoking gun, some plant or group of them that would clearly explain much of the owner's allergies. In the backyard I found it: Growing in the corner of the yard, hanging over their large wooden jacuzzi, was a huge fruitless mulberry tree. These "litter-free" mulberry trees are all male clones, and in springtime this one would shed hundreds of billions of highly allergenic tiny pollen grains. Everything and everyone below it would be showered in pollen.

Weeks, even months after this huge male tree had dropped its entire noxious load, much of this pollen would still be lying around, on the deck, on the patio chairs, on the barbeque. The mulberry pollen would be on the wooden walkway to the house, and plenty of pollen would be tracked into the house daily. I recommended that they either give the tree a sex change – cut back the tree hard and then top-graft it to scion wood from a female mulberry tree – or just cut it down.

When we went inside for a cup of coffee I was feeling pretty confident about having solved their worst problems. I had my coffee and then, just as I was walking out of the house, I noticed several very large indoor Umbrella Trees (*Schefflera* species) growing in a big planter box below a skylight in their living room. They looked dry, as though they needed a good drink of water. I took a closer look, and they were indeed very dry. They were also literally dripping with scale, whiteflies, and mold.

My last recommendation was this: Take an antihistamine and then put on some old clothes with long sleeves and a facemask; rip these Umbrella Trees out, haul them outside, and stuff them in the trash containers; cover the containers, go back inside and clean everything, then immediately take a shower and put the old clothes in the wash.

I thought I'd found the smoking gun – the male junipers in the front and the male mulberry in the back – but had almost missed the worst offender right in the middle of their house!

I find prime examples of out of whack, sexually manipulated, highly allergenic landscapes everywhere I turn. Once you know what to look for you can see it all too clearly. This toxic landscaping is by no means confined to home landscapes. A few years ago I was giving a series of lectures at the Anaheim Home and Garden Show, near Disneyland. The show put my wife, Yvonne, and me up across the street at a rather swank hotel (one of the nicer perks of being a writer).

We were sitting in the jacuzzi, and I noticed growing next to and above us in large cement planters a great many Gold Dust Plants (*Aucuba japonica*). I knew these were all separate-sexed plants, and just for fun I asked Yvonne to go off to our left and see how many she could find that had the tell-tale red berries of female *Aucuba* plants. These bright red female fruits are the size of small cherries and are hard to miss.

Yvonne went off and started looking one way, and I went the other. In all we counted over two hundred of these Gold Dust Plants. And how many berries did we find? None. All the plants were males. In the springtime when these landscape shrubs would be in bloom, all of them would be producing plenty of allergenic pollen. *Aucuba* pollen is relatively heavy, but since these were in raised beds, the pollen would easily fall on the guests below as they soaked in the hot tub or lounged around the pool. Perhaps some of them would blame their itchy noses and eyes on too much chlorine in the pool?

How does this sort of thing happen so often? How have our landscapes become so often predominantly male and so remarkably allergenic? These are some of the questions I have long been asking, and here in *Safe Sex in the Garden*, we'll explore together the answers.

Plant Sex and Allergies

Plant sex and allergies are intimately connected. Without an understanding of plant sex, we'll continue to suffer far too much from pollen allergies. Pollen itself is, of course, the essence of the male parts of plants; it's the plant's equivalent of a male animal's semen. The female part of a plant is called the *pistil,* and it's where the male pollen settles and sticks. At the base of the pistil are the *ovaries* (or *ovules*) where the seeds eventually form.

Male trees produce pollen and female trees do not. But female trees produce seeds or fruit and are often considered messy. And therein lies the rub. Because male trees don't produce "litter," landscapers plant male trees, millions of them. With each passing year female trees become more rare. The results? Pollen, lots and lots of pollen, and an ever-growing number of people with allergies, asthma, and other pollen-caused illnesses.

Plant Sex in History

In 1676 the English physician Sir Thomas Millington first discovered that plants have a sex life. Botanist Konrad Sprengel first wrote about dioecious (separate-sexed) plants and their abundant production of pollen in 1812. But in the puritanical climate of the early 1800s and in the late 1600s when Millington discovered plants' sex lives, it was considered lewd to speak or write of such things. Many botanical writers went to great lengths to avoid any words connected to sex, even avoiding using words such as "pollen." Even the great plant geneticist Gregor Mendel (1822–84) and the pioneering naturalist Charles Darwin (1809–82) were both purposefully vague and obscure on floral sexual matters. However, our greatest botanist, Karl Linnaeus (1707–78), was no such prude. Linnaeus based his entire revolutionary system of plant and animal classification, *binomial nomenclature* (genus, species), on the flora or fauna's sexual parts. (By the way, "genus" means "group," and "species" means "kind." For example, in the case of *Malus domestica,* "*Malus*" is Latin for "apple" and "*domestica*" tells us what kind of apple it is – domesticated.)

That some plants were male and others female was actually understood by some long before the 1600s. In ancient times marauding tribes would sometimes cut down or burn all the "bull" palms in their enemy's date orchards. They realized that with no male trees to pollinate the female palm trees, there would be no dates. Since only one male was needed for every fifty females, it was easier to just kill off all the males than it was to kill the entire orchard. And as far as ruining future crops of dates, it was just as effective.

The overabundance of male trees in our cities today is one result of all this prudence. As absurd as it sounds, I have found that many of the growers who propagate these male trees are not even aware that they are male. They simply think they are "seedless." Likewise, few of the landscapers and homeowners who buy and plant all these allergy-causing male trees realize that they are male. Again, they think that they're just planting low-maintenance "fruit-less" trees. They rarely think of the sex involved. Even our botanists prefer to stick to the terms *staminate* and *pistillate,* rather than simply saying male and female. I, however, prefer to use the perfectly understandable words "male" and "female." It would seem that the sexual revolution of the '60s somehow was missed by many in botany and horticulture.

Recent Progress and New Data

My own take on plant sexuality is different than that of the botanists and geneticists. I am chiefly interested in how plant sex affects our own everyday health. A little bit of pollen is almost never a problem, but today we are literally bombarded with this biopollutant. Our modern landscapes actually are killing us, killing many thousands of us each year. Close to seven thousand people die each year from sudden death caused by asthma, and a great many of these deaths are pollen triggered. Recent European studies have found that death rates rise significantly on days with peak pollen counts.[1] In addition, millions of people are made miserable with allergies, asthma, and other respiratory-related illnesses. If foreign enemies did this to us, we'd declare war on them.

When I set out to write this book, I decided from the start that I wanted something new that would shake people up. For too long now I have been aware of the rampant apathy and ignorance surrounding the issues of urban pollen. I wanted to dig deeper into certain areas, and to use this book both as a vehicle for sharing recent discoveries and, more importantly, as a catalyst for social change. I am most grateful for the warm response my work has received from so many magazine and newspaper health, environment, and garden editors. However, a few reviewers of my work have deemed it "too political." "Too political?" I need to get even more political. Massive numbers of people are getting sick and thousands are dying for the cause of tidy sidewalks. If I must be political in order to get something done, so be it.

My research has generated a rather amazing amount of press, and there have been full-page lead articles on it in many newspapers. But in several articles, reporters came up with some local "expert" who hadn't seen my book and who dismissed my work out of hand.

"What you plant in your own yard doesn't make any difference," these naysayers wrote. "Pollen can blow in from hundreds of miles away, so whatever you have in your own yard makes no difference at all."

These local "experts" are dead wrong. What you plant in your own yard can make all the difference in the world. Simply put, if you plant your own yard full of heavy pollen-producing, high-allergy plants, you'll be getting all that pollen on a regular basis. It's much like living with someone who smokes cigarettes in your house versus occasionally passing a smoker on the street. It's all a question of degree.

David Stadtner, M.D., the Stockton, California, allergist who wrote the foreword to my book *Allergy-Free Gardening*, recently wrote in a letter to the editor of the *Star-Ledger* in Newark, New Jersey, "I have had many patients whose allergy symptoms improved by removing an offending tree or shrub near their home." But do we really need doctors or horticulturists to tell us this? Just plain old common sense, isn't it?

It was just as obvious to me that I needed to write *Safe Sex in the Garden* in order to clear up all the misinformation and confusion that exists about the direct connections between plant sex and illness.

Many allergists understand that if someone is allergic to, say, six things and three of them are removed, then he or she may become symptom free. This is an important insight. By creating an allergy-free yard you will have eliminated the closest, most intense sources of what ails you. Even though your body will contact some allergens from outside your own area of control, your symptoms will diminish and sometimes disappear.

How Full Is Your Bucket?

Another way of thinking about the cause of allergies is through the analogy of the bucket. When you get up in the morning and feel great, you have an "empty bucket." Then perhaps you absent-mindedly run your hand over the top of the TV, kicking up a small dose of quickly inhaled dust. The dust goes in your empty bucket.

At breakfast you may eat something you're allergic to, and that too goes in your bucket. At this point you probably feel perfectly fine. You then inhale a dose of pollen from the bouquet of daisies on the table. This goes in your bucket too. But there is still room in your bucket and you still feel great. Your cat walks by and you inhale some cat dander. It goes in your now quickly filling bucket, but still, you're all right.

Now you go outside to get the newspaper, and a little puff of wind knocks a small cloud of invisible pollen from the seedless male tree overhead. You inhale this pollen-filled air, and those thousands of allergens go in your almost-full bucket. Suddenly it overflows, and now you feel miserable.

It is usually the cumulative effect of multiple allergens that makes us feel lousy. The trick is not to let our buckets overflow, that is, to eliminate and avoid as many likely allergens as possible. We need not eliminate all the allergens in our environments, just some of them. As with so many things, allergy is usually a question of degree. In the above case, with some safe sex in your garden, you would have remained symptom free.

Recent Progress

Despite much recent progress, I am impatient and wish it would happen faster. At the request of parents, I visited two elementary schools recently to evaluate the school landscapes. Of twenty-six trees at one school, I found fifteen highly allergenic male Yew Pines and six even more allergenic male Chinese Pistache trees. Out of seventeen trees at the second school, fifteen of them were extremely allergenic, large male "fruitless" mulberry trees. I found no female trees at either school. Springtime pollen levels at these two schools must be incredible. Sadly these schools are in no way exceptions.

Years ago America's dentists took the lead in prevention of cavities by urging that small amounts of fluoride be used in drinking water. This is now a widespread and efficient practice. I hope allergists and nurserypeople will follow the dentists' good example and urge an end to the use of all these highly allergenic landscape plants. Social responsibility requires no less.

On the bright side, many groups of gardeners have been working hard to educate city planners, landscapers, and other gardeners. They have welcomed me with open arms. I have given numerous talks to interested, knowledgeable, socially involved groups such as local and state garden clubs and Master Gardeners. Speaking to audiences of gardeners is always a real pleasure for me. They know and love and appreciate plants. They ask intelligent questions and are always eager to learn new things. Some gardeners have been insisting that their landscapers too understand how plant sex relates to pollen allergies. Gardeners have been insisting that their local nurseries stock more female plants. Some gardeners have been going to city council meetings and to homeowner associations and insisting that the rights of those with allergies be respected. Some local pollen control ordinances already exist and more are being discussed and will hopefully soon be enacted. I have been planting the seeds of social change with these talks, and the gardeners are fertile ground. The rebellion has already begun.

I encourage anyone who doesn't already belong to a garden club to join one or to become a Master Gardener, or better yet, to do both. Garden club members and Master Gardeners are wonderful, smart, enthusiastic, socially responsible people. They help to make our world a friendlier and more beautiful place. I encourage all of you to help. Write letters to magazine and newspaper editors; talk to your own landscapers or gardeners; talk to the people at the nurseries; ask horticulture, landscape, and design professors to teach that our health will be directly affected by what we plant. Talk to your doctors about it, talk to your friends, just do something.

As I said earlier I have occasionally been accused of being "too political," but getting results often does boil down to politics. I ask all my readers to get involved. I especially encourage all of you with allergies, or those of you with loved ones who have allergies or other breathing problems, to stand up for your rights. You have a perfect right to air that isn't filled with excessive amounts of pollen. The trees and shrubs and lawns that cities, states, parks, and counties plant have a profound effect on your health. Insist that those in charge always seriously consider your health when choosing what flowers, shrubs, and trees to plant.

As we explore how plant sexuality in our immediate green environment affects our health and well-being, I hope you'll find *Safe Sex in the Garden* to be both a helpful companion in your own gardening as well as a call to action. Together we can make our communities and our world a healthier place to live.

To those who may have stumbled onto this book seeking more erotic reading, sorry, you're out of luck. To the rest of you, a hearty welcome! May all your gardens be beautiful, fun, mellow, healthy, and of course, very sexy.

CHAPTER I

The Gardener Who Always Talks about Sex

As I said earlier I've been giving lots of talks the past few years, and along the way I seem to have picked up the reputation as the gardener who always talks about sex. Often I speak immediately after everyone has just finished a huge lunch, and sex, I've found, is one topic that wakes people up. But actually I do need to talk about sex – plant sex at any rate. It is, after all, common misunderstandings about plant sex that have created much of this current allergy epidemic. Let's hope we can clear up some of this sexual confusion and in the process take more control over our own personal airspace.

In this chapter I will explain in detail exactly how we ended up with an explosion of urban pollen, and we'll explore some other often-proposed reasons for the surge of allergy and asthma. Some of these reasons make sense, and others are patently absurd. I think my all time "favorite" cause for this was the doctor who blamed it all on women's lib! More on this in a moment.

An Allergy Epidemic

You doubt there really is an allergy epidemic? A few figures then:

- As late as 1959 it was widely reported that allergy affected only between 2 and 5 percent of the United States population.

- By 1985 most estimates of allergy put it at 12 to 15 percent of the United States population.

- By December 1999 the American College of Asthma, Allergy and Immunology reported that allergy had jumped yet again. Some 38 percent of us now suffered from allergies.

An increase from 2 to 5 percent up to almost 40 percent in my own lifetime is an incredible rise in allergies. Perhaps some of this surge can be attributed to doctors becoming more aware of allergies and to better diagnosis. But this can in no way explain away such a tremendous leap in numbers of people affected. The skin tests normally used in allergy determination are not much different from what they were forty years ago.

AN EPIDEMIC OF HOUSE DUST?

Some writers claim that house dust is the culprit, but seriously, are our houses so much dustier now than ever before? Some suggest they are. My brother-in-law, a college professor, once went to a famous doctor, and while being examined he tried to tell the doc about my book. "Look," said the doctor, "you want to know why there's so much allergy these days?"

"Sure," said my brother-in-law.

"Women's lib," said the doctor. "All these women had to go out there and compete with men. They had to have everything – family, house, job, kids. They don't keep their houses clean anymore, they're filthy, and that's why we have so much allergy now."

Personally, I don't buy it. I have seen plenty of immaculate, dust-free houses where both the parents and the kids suffered from allergies. I hardly think we can blame all of this on more dust, much less on women's lib.

AN EPIDEMIC OF CLEANLINESS?

Another theory going round these days is that we have so much allergy now because people are too clean. Their home environments lack enough allergens to keep their immune systems charged. This is one theory that may have merit. What is interesting in particular about this common theory is that it is the exact opposite of the explanation that we have so much more house dust now.

There may well be something to the new idea that overuse of antibacterial soaps causes problems. It is quite possible that we can get too clean. We should be aiming to limit allergens in our environment, not to eradicate them. A low level of allergens will build up our immune systems. Statistics consistently show that children raised on farms, around animals, have fewer allergies than those raised in squeaky clean urban households.

AN EPIDEMIC OF COCKROACHES?

This theory keeps coming up all the time too. Exposure to cockroaches and their allergenic insect dander causes allergies. Okay, I'll buy that. But claims that we have far more exposure to cockroaches now than in the past? This would appear to be an overreach. There are no statistics that show any kind of increase in numbers of cockroaches. Newer houses are built tighter than older ones and have fewer roaches. However, in some inner city areas where the buildings are rundown, roaches and their dander are serious problems. For the typical middle-class asthma allergy sufferer though, this is not the case.

In the 1950s and 1960s, and in some areas even into the 1970s, as Dutch Elm disease killed off almost all of the American Elm street trees we used to see everywhere, new methods of landscaping took hold.

The elms were perfect flowered (with male and female parts in the same flowers), insect pollinated, and shed only small amounts of pollen. The elms caused a certain low amount of allergy, but nothing compared to what has been caused by their replacements. Their replacements in most cases were high pollen-producing, wind-pollinated trees, and a huge number of these were male clones.

So what's the problem with male clones?

Pollen. Male trees all produce pollen, lots of pollen, and airborne pollen at that. All male trees will produce allergenic pollen, and this pollen will cause allergies, asthma, rash, sinus conditions, headaches, fatigue, irritability, and many other serious health problems. It was recently reported in a pioneering report in the British medical journal *The Lancet* that deaths increased on days with peak pollen counts.[1] Deaths from heart attack rose 5 percent, deaths from heart disease were up 6 percent, deaths from COPD (a group of pulmonary/lung diseases) increased 15 percent, and pneumonia deaths jumped 17 percent. Most of the pollen involved in these particular studies came from grasses and birch and poplar trees, but many allergy researchers, myself included, believe that any species of pollen is potentially problematic. Excessive pollen levels are simply not healthy.

Unfortunately, since the 1950s, it has also become common practice to cut down seedling trees once it's determined that they're female – since they are deemed "messy." Seedling male trees are generally left to grow old and large. This "unnatural selection" has taken a large toll on the females and has left us with ever more urban pollen. Between specifically planting large numbers of male clones and the systematic removal of female trees, we have created quite a situation. As is so often the case, when we manipulate large ecosystems and don't consider the consequences, we create a host of new problems.

Horticulturists knew that female plants produced seeds, seed-pods, and fruit. This "litter" fell on the sidewalks and created a "mess." By using only *asexually propagated* (no sex involved) *cultivars* (culti-vated varieties), they were able to create "litter-free" landscapes. These trees required less maintenance and were (and still are) very popular with city arborists and the public. In the United States to-day, four of the five top-selling street tree cultivars are male clones.

Female *(pistillate)* flowers on female trees or shrubs (with their roots grounded in the earth) produce a negative electrical current. Their hundreds of thousands of *stigmas* at the tips of the pistils are broad and sticky. Airborne pollen from male plants is light and dry, and it picks up a positive electrical impulse as it tumbles about in the air. Because of the + and – electrical charges the pollen and the stigmas are drawn to each other. They are mutually attractive. Mother Nature saw to it that pollen would land, and stick, exactly where it was needed. Female plants are nature's pollen traps, our natural air cleaners.

Today, though, most of the female plants are long gone from our urban landscapes. Female trees produce no pollen, zero; they are pollen-free trees, but they are scarce in our city landscapes. The pollen from the males floats about, seeking a moist, sticky, elec-trically charged target. We humans emit an electrical charge, and our mucous membranes, our eyes, skin, and especially the linings of our nose and throat, now trap this wayward pollen. We have be-come the targets.

SO, WHAT EXACTLY IS THE PROBLEM?

The problem is that landscapers, city planners, schools, and homeowners all wanted these "litter-free" landscapes. They planted millions of trees they called "fruitless" or "seedless," that is, male trees. As such they don't drop any messy seeds on the sidewalks. Instead they pump tons of highly allergenic pollen into the air.

Pollen is the invisible littler. A typical pollen grain is about twenty microns in diameter, small enough to pass right through the tightest window screen. I recently shook some pollen from a male yew onto a glass slide, placed a small square of window screen over the slide, and then looked at it with my microscope. I wanted to see how much protection, if any, a screen actually was. Although I knew what to expect, I was nonetheless amazed at what I saw. I would estimate that as many as a thousand grains of this pollen could simultaneously pass through each tiny square in the window screen!

Pollen all over our sidewalks may not be as noticeable as seed or old fruit from female trees, but it is there and it does cause allergies. It is litter and it does make millions of people sick.

What Are We to Do?

Well, if you're reading this now, you are headed in the right direction. You'll soon be part of the solution because to make a difference the most important element of all will be education.

Back to sex. The first step is learning how to tell the boys from the girls.

I get a lot of email from people asking me how to tell what the sex of a plant is. "Am I supposed to turn it upside down and take a close look?" is one that I'm asked all the time.

No! It's not quite that simple.

With some species of plants it is easy to determine the sex, but with others it takes someone trained in botany. One of the aims of this book is to make it a great deal easier for you to determine a plant's sex. And which sex is it we want to see used more in our gardens and landscapes? Females! More females. Feminists, we need you!

As I mentioned earlier, in the past decade four of the top five most used street trees in the United States were male clones. We need to reverse this trend. When society values tidy sidewalks and litter-free lawns over clean fresh air, it's time for a change.

The Birds and the Bees, and the Butterflies Too

Male trees produce no fruit for birds and small animals to eat, and they usually produce little or no nectar for the butterflies, hummingbirds, and honeybees. The last three decades of sterile, litter-free landscapes have dramatically reduced urban food sources for many of nature's small creatures. As the sale of wind-pollinated, male-cloned street trees expanded, it was accompanied by the decline in numbers of the cities' butterflies and honeybees. Deprived of major early-season food sources, many of these species simply starved. Allergy-free gardens and landscapes, with their reliance on female and insect-pollinated plants, may indeed be a bit messier. But they will also bring us less allergy, less asthma, cleaner air, and more birds, honeybees, and butterflies.

Your Health

In the past twenty years or so the concept of urban forests and of urban forestry has been growing. It is an idea that makes plenty of sense too, because inside our cities, the city trees are indeed our forests, and they have a powerful effect on our quality of life. The undergrowth of these urban forests is made up of our shrubs, vines, hedges, perennials, annuals, and our large expanses of ground covers and lawns.

All the plants growing in a city, along with the insects, birds, and all the other creatures living in them, form a large ecosystem. The makeup and health of the entire urban forest ecosystem strongly affect both our mental and physical health. Likewise, the choices we make and the care we put into the upkeep of our urban forests also have a profound affect on the health of the entire ecosystem, ourselves included.

People like to say, "Without your health, you don't have anything." Just how true is this?

Think about the last time that you were really sick. When we are seriously ill we are no longer interested in making more money, in fishing, golfing, sailing, hiking, canoeing, biking, surfing, reading, movies, good music. Shoot, when we're really sick we aren't interested in good food or even in sex.

So, just because we may feel perfectly well today, let's not forget just how wonderful it is to feel good, to be healthy. Let's do everything we can to be healthy, including practicing safe sex in our gardens. As any honest person can tell you, too many males always spells trouble!

Okay then, please do read on, and from me to you, a toast: "Here's to your good health!"

More about Sex— Some Terms to Learn

In order to fully understand plant sex and how it relates to our health, we need to first understand some of the basic lingo.

So, are all plants either male or female? No, not at all. Some of them are separate sexed, but by no means all of them. Let's explore the most basic flowering systems quickly. You probably won't remember all of this on first reading. That's fine. Just come back later to chapter 2 and look it over if you get mixed up on the terms down the road.

Pistils and Stamens

The main female part of the flower is the *pistil*. On the tip of the pistil is the *stigma,* and it is here that pollen settles and sticks. Down at the base of the pistil are the *ovaries* (or *ovules*), where the seeds

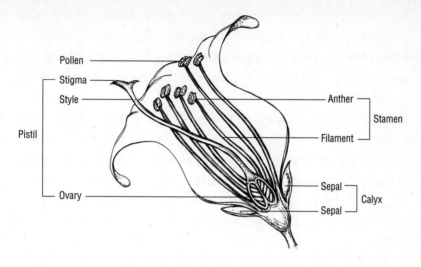

Parts of a perfect flower.

will eventually form. A separate-sexed plant that is all female, one that has no male flowers on it at all, is what botanists call a "pistil-late" plant.

The main male parts of a flower are the *stamens.* On the tip of each stamen is the *anther,* which holds a large collection of pollen. A flower that has only stamens and no female parts is called a "sta-minate" flower. Likewise, a separate-sexed (dioecious) plant that is all male and has no female flowers is also called a staminate plant.

Dioecious-Flowered, or Separate-Sexed, Plants

These dioecious plants, which may be annuals, perennials, grasses, shrubs, vines, or trees, are totally separate sexed. This may at first seem quite odd to many readers, but certain individual plants, just like individual people, are only one sex. The sexual characteristics of a plant are not all that different than those of a human. Females produce seeds or eggs, and males produce pollen or semen. Pollen from male plants is simply the plant's version of semen, and up close, the pollen-filled anthers on the tips of the male stamens look remarkably like miniature scrotums. Considering that huge amounts of allergy and asthma are directly caused by excessive wind-blown pollen, it might not be too far-fetched to say that pollen allergy is no doubt the most common sexually transmitted disease in the world.

With a dioecious species of tree, a willow for example, all of the willow trees will be either male trees or female trees. With all separate-sexed species of plants, the males will produce pollen-bearing stamens but no seeds. The females will produce fertile ovules (eggs) in their female flowers but no pollen. If a female flower is pollinated with pollen from a male plant, it will then produce fruit and seeds.

If a separate-sexed plant has seeds or fruit on it, it is always a female plant. If it never makes any seeds or fruit, it is probably a male. Some examples of dioecious plants are asparagus, Red Maples, Box Elders, junipers, yews, hollies, ash, poplars, Date Palms, poison ivy, poison oak, and pepper trees.

Monoecious, or Two-Sexed, Plants

A monoecious plant has many male and female flowers, so it is both a male and female plant. Individual flowers on monoecious plants will be unisexual – that is, they will be either male flowers or female flowers – but both sexes will be present on the same plant. A good example of a monoecious plant is the pine tree. On the ends of the branches will be clusters of male flowers (cones of pollen), and farther back in the tree will be female flowers, which will turn into pinecones. Most monoecious-flowered plants, like the dioecious ones, are pollinated by the wind. Corn is another good example of a monoecious plant. The tops of the corn plants, the tassels, are the male pollen-bearing flowers. Lower down on the plant, the ears of corn, they are actually clusters of female flowers. Other examples of monoecious plants are begonias, cucumbers, cypress, birch, oaks, pecans, walnuts, and watermelons. Not all monoecious plants cause allergies, but a great many highly allergenic trees are wind pollinated and monoecious flowered.

Perfect-Flowered Plants

A perfect-flowered plant, like a rose or an apple tree, will have fertile flowers where the female parts (the pistil) are usually in the middle, and the male parts (the stamens) are also in the same flower and usually surround the female. Sometimes the stamens will be shorter than the pistil, as in a perfect-flowered fuchsia. The reverse can also be true, as in the perfect-flowered apricot blossom, where the stamens rise above the pistil. There are always multiples of stamens in a perfect flower, but numbers of pistils will vary. In a single-seeded plum blossom there is but one pistil, but in a multiseeded apple the pistil may be tipped with multiple stigmas.

The pollen from the stamens doesn't have far to go to reach the female pistil. As a result perfect-flowered plants usually cause less allergy – but not always!

Most perfect-flowered plants are pollinated by honeybees, bumblebees, certain flies, moths, and even occasionally by hummingbirds and bats. Some common perfect-flowered plants are strawberries, lilies, tulips, tomatoes, pears, peaches, and magnolias.

Polygamous Plants

Polygamous flowering plants will have both perfect flowers and single-sexed flowers on the same plant. A buckeye tree is a good example of polygamous flowering. The buckeye in bloom will have great clusters of flowers on the ends of each branch. Often these clusters will be a foot or more in length. On the tips of the flowering branches, all the blooms are perfect flowers, each individual flower complete with fertile female and male sex organs.

FOUR MAIN TYPES OF FLOWERING SYSTEMS

Dioecious, or separate sexed	Only the males have pollen.
Monoecious	Separate unisexual (one-sex) flowers, both male and female, and both are present on the same plant.
Perfect flowered	Every flower on the plant has both male and female parts in the same flower.
Polygamous flowered	Have perfect-flowered flowers *and* have unisexual flowers, all on the same plant.

However, six inches below the tips of the branch there will be many unisexual (one-sex) flowers, and with buckeye these will always be male-only flowers. The clusters of buckeye flowers are designed by nature to be pollinated by both insect and the wind, and as a result pollen from the male-only flowers indeed can become airborne and cause allergy.

However, sometimes a polygamous tree will have an assortment of perfect flowers and unisexual all-female flowers. This is often seen with certain varieties of persimmons. A tree like this is almost always entirely insect pollinated, will shed virtually no pollen, and so poses little allergy risk.

Top-Grafting, Sex Changes

In some cases existing male trees can be *top-grafted* with *scion wood* from a female tree of the same species (see illustration on page 24).

This will effect a sex change. Some years ago I was talking to a city arborist (who was from the Midwest) about how his city had such an incredible number of male-cloned street trees. Most of these were recently planted, highly allergenic, male Chinese Pistache trees. I told him that since these were fairly young trees, and since they were all deciduous, that it would be a good idea to top-graft them all over to female. He could do this in the winter when they were dormant. (Deciduous trees are far easier to bud or graft than evergreen trees since they have a dormant season. A dormant tree has no leaves – through which water is lost – so a dormant graft is much less likely to dry out and fail.) "You should give them all a sex change," I said.

The arborist shook his head and looked dismayed. "That is so California," he said.

Perhaps it was, but I'd much rather graft a male tree to female than chop it down. I've top-grafted quite a few fruitless male mulberry trees. They're also deciduous and go dormant in the winter. Every mulberry I grafted took. In one season those highly allergenic male trees were converted into allergy-free female trees.

Clones and Cultivars

Readers often get confused about the terms "clone" and "cultivar." With trees these words mean much the same thing. A cultivar is simply a cultivated variety, propagated (produced) asexually by grafting, budding, layering, cuttings, or tissue culture. There are cultivated varieties, or "cloned," male and female trees.

Each cloned tree or shrub will have a common name, a Latin name, and a specific cultivar name. For example: Red Maple, *Acer rubrum,* 'Davey Red.' Red Maple is the common name, *Acer rubrum* is the Latin name, and 'Davey Red' is the cultivar (clone) name. Every single tree of Red Maple, *Acer rubrum,* 'Davey Red' is cloned from the same original tree. Since in this case the original tree was a female maple, so are all of its clones.

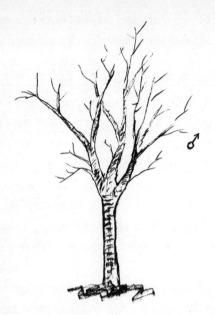

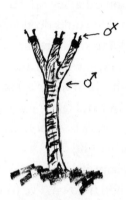

A. Dormant deciduous male tree before top-grafting.

B. Male tree cut back to three main branches and two scions of female wood cleft-grafted on each. (Two scions are used on each branch to increase the odds of a good take.)

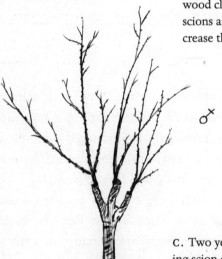

C. Two years later, the strongest growing scion on each graft has been kept and the weaker one removed.

Congratulations!

Congratulations – you've just completed the official Ogren plant sex education course (abbreviated version)! Understanding the four flowering systems won't be absolutely necessary to understand the rest of *Safe Sex in the Garden,* but it will help. If this is all new to you, it's possible that you may be feeling a bit overwhelmed and confused. Don't worry about it – chances are you aren't the only one. If you don't understand the systems yet, read the chapter over, several times if need be. If you've done that and are still mixed up, email me (see page 213) and let me know what's confusing you.

Other more complex and obscure flowering systems, which are less common than those explained above, do exist, but we won't even go there – unless, of course, you want some extra credit!

CHAPTER 3

How to Tell the Boys from the Girls

M ale plants are nothing but guaranteed trouble for anyone with allergies. Actually male plants are guaranteed trouble for everyone, since given enough overexposure to abundant pollen, it appears that almost anyone can develop an allergy.

What if you go to a nursery and you want to buy some pollen-free female plants? How do you know which ones to buy? Or perhaps you are in your own backyard, looking at your own existing landscape. How do you know the sex of these plants? In this chapter, we'll learn how to sex plants.

Plants from Nurseries

If you are buying plants at a nursery, especially trees or shrubs, don't buy them unless they are properly tagged. The tag should have the common name, the complete Latin name of the plant, with genus and species, and the plant's cultivar name. For example, with the Red Maple often just called 'October Glory,' the correct tag would read, in this precise order: Red Maple, *Acer rubrum,* 'October Glory.' It also might be listed accurately but a tad differently such as *Acer rubrum* c (or cv, or CV) 'October Glory.' The c or CV simply stands for "cultivar," which is the horticultural version of a cloned plant.

It would also be smart to actually have in your hand a copy of *Allergy-Free Gardening,* so that you could compare for yourself the exact name of the plant in the nursery with the exact same plant in the book. If the plant is not named and ranked in the book, it's safest not to buy it. If I was unclear as to the sex of a particular cultivar, I either noted this fact or did not include that cultivar in my writing. When looking over a tree or shrub in a container at a nursery, you'll have to compare the genus, the species, *and* the common name with what is in my book to be sure of getting a pollen-free female plant.

Let me give you a few examples of some confusion on this subject so that you can avoid mistakes. Several years ago, just prior to the publication of *Allergy-Free Gardening,* I was asked to select all the plant materials for a new low-pollen landscape that was being installed at the "Breathe Easy Office" of the American Lung Association in Richmond, Virginia. The landscape designer had already installed a row of Himalayan Junipers. Someone at the nursery where she bought these plants had told her they were female because they had berries on them.

Now, most species of juniper are dioecious, separate-sexed, and berries are indeed an indication of femaleness in a separate-sexed species. However, Himalayan Junipers, which are monoecious (both sexes on the same plant, remember?), are the exception. I had to recommend that they pull up all of these plants, repot them, and return them to the nursery. They were replaced with female junipers.

There was a second bit of sexual confusion with plants in this same landscape. I visited the American Lung Association in

Richmond, Virginia, again in spring of 2002 to give a talk, and to my horror there in our wonderful low-pollen landscape was a whole row of pollen-laden male yews in full bloom! We tracked down the problem, and the plants were soon removed. I mention this here because it is an example of exactly why one needs to have a copy of *Allergy-Free Gardening* in hand at the nursery to know with certainty, which plants will be pollen-free and which will not be.

In the case of the Lung Association low-pollen landscape, a dozen yews, all tagged (incorrectly) as *Taxus × media* 'Densiformis,' had been planted because, again, someone told the designer that this variety was always female. I purposely did not include 'Densiformis' in my book because I had discovered that in the trade the variety is often confused. One nursery will sell a male yew calling it 'Densiformis' while another will sell the correct, original female one. The original 'Densiformis' yew had indeed been a female clone, but gardeners could no longer count on this. What had happened was that over time some propagator had taken cuttings from a male yew, had grown them and then sold them, labeling them incorrectly as 'Densiformis.' These plants were grown, and eventually someone else rooted cuttings from these incorrectly named plants and again tagged them as 'Densiformis.' This sort of cultivar confusion has occurred with a number of plants.

When I visited an arboretum I made note of all cultivars grown there as to the exact sex of each one. When I visited other arboretums, I compared notes. I also visited many nurseries and compared cultivars being sold with my original notes. If there was any discrepancy, I considered the cultivar "confused" or not reliable, that is, one that I could not safely ever recommend as being female. The cultivars I have identified in *Allergy-Free Gardening* as female are only the ones that are consistently the same.

If there were books besides my own that consistently listed the sex of most individual nursery plants, I would gladly recommend them to you here, but unfortunately there are not any other such books. With a few species of plants, such as holly, many horticulture books will list the sex, but this is limited to very few species and is always the exception to the rule. In my books the sex of a plant may not always be mentioned, but each plant cultivar will always have an OPALS™ ranking. OPALS is an acronym for the Ogren Plant-Allergy Scale – a scheme of rank I designed to measure a plant's level of allergy potential. OPALS ranks range from 1 to 10, 1 being the least allergenic, 10 the most allergenic. A plant need not necessarily be female to be allergy-free, and a good OPALS ranking is always an indication of low potential to cause allergy or asthma.

I do answer personal emails, so if you can't get the information you need from your nursery professionals or from this book or *Allergy-Free Gardening*, please write me, care of my website, www.allergyfree-gardening.com.

When considering a plant, talk to your nursery personnel and ask them about the sex of a plant in question. (Quite a few nursery professionals have read *Allergy-Free Gardening* themselves, many of them have heard me speak, and some have even taken classes from me.) They ought to be able to sex the plants for you.

Plants Already in Your Yard

In your yard, you want to look for (and hope to find!) fruit, seeds, and/or seedpods. By "seeds" I mean seeds such as the long, thin ones you would see on a female ash tree, or the winged seeds on a female Red Maple, or the hard nuts produced by a hazelnut bush. The term "seedpods" would include all those seed-filled pods from pod-forming shrubs, vines, and trees. These seed-bearing vessels may be long and fuzzy (such as the pods of a wisteria vine), long and smooth-sided (such as the pods found on a female Honey Locust tree), or flat and rounded (like the pods on a jacaranda tree). By "fruit" I mean any sort of plant-produced fleshy fruit or berry, not just edible fruits like apples or oranges. A rose hip is a fruit, as

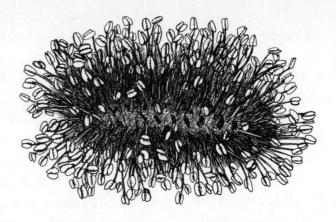

Male (pollen) flowers on a male willow tree.

are the red berries of a hawthorn or a *Pyracantha* or a *Cotoneaster*. Now, just because a plant has fruit on it doesn't mean for sure that it is a female (it could be perfect-flowered or monoecious), *but* if it does have fruit or seeds or seedpods you can be certain that it is *not* a male plant. Remember, male plants produce no seeds, seedpods, or fruit and are nothing but guaranteed trouble for anyone with allergies.

But what if it is the wrong time of year and there aren't any fruits on your plants? Must you then use a different strategy?

When I asked how to tell if a plant was male, a professor once told me, "Just look and see if it has any pollen on it." That advice was not nearly as good as it might have seemed. Male plants don't produce pollen all year round. (Thank goodness!) Sometimes you just cannot tell the sex of a tree or shrub in your yard, particularly in late fall or during wintertime when many trees and shrubs are dormant. In this case you may have to wait until springtime when you can look at the flowers.

Male flowers will indeed have pollen, but bear in mind that pollen is not always that easy to see, nor is it always bright yellow. I've seen pollen that was white, gray, green, brown, red, and even purple. Nonetheless once a tree is blooming, it is entirely possible to sex it.

Gender Giveaways

Below is a quick list of some of the more commonly sold and used landscape shrubs, trees, and ground covers that are dioecious (separate-sexed). These species will include the male plants you'll want most to avoid as well as the finest pollen-free female plants available. Here's what to look for to tell those boys from the girls.

Alpine Currant, _Ribes alpinum_. Some types of currants, such as the hardy, deciduous shrub Alpine Currant, only produce the small, bright red fruits on the female bushes.

Ash trees, _Fraxinus_ species. Ash trees, if female, will have small flowers that look like the winged seeds that will appear after flowering. Female ash trees usually produce many seeds that hang on the trees long into the summer.

Cedar trees, _Cedrus_ species. Female cedar trees produce large, fat, rounded cones that stand 4 inches tall, upright on the branches. The cones on male cedars are much smaller, less than half as large as the cones on the female cedar trees. Do not confuse cedars with junipers, as is often done. They're two totally different species.

Coyote Brush or Coyote Bush, _Baccharis_ species. With the landscape ragweed relative, the ground cover Coyote Brush (_Baccharis_ species), the female plants make large amounts of fluffy, cottonlike seeds. The "litter-free" male plants just produce that "invisible litter," allergenic pollen.

Fringe Tree, _Chionanthus_ species. Female Fringe Trees make small, olivelike, hard green fruits that turn almost black by fall. Males make no fruit at all.

Ginkgo biloba. Only the female _Ginkgo_ trees make the green, golfball-sized fruits. The large seeds inside these fruits (ginkgo nuts) are very tasty, but the juice of the smelly fleshy fruit can cause a nasty contact skin rash, so handle with care.

Gold Dust Plant, *Aucuba japonica*. Females of these colorful shrubs produce thumbnail-sized bright red fruits. Males make none.

Hardy Rubber Trees, *Eucommia ulmoides*; tallow trees, *Sapium* species; *Hovenia*; *Mallotus*; *Sapindus*; *Idesia*; and *Cudrania*. Hardy Rubber Trees *(Eucommia ulmoides),* tallow trees *(Sapium* species), and other separate-sexed landscape trees such as *Hovenia, Mallotus, Sapindus, Idesia,* and *Cudrania* only have their small, long-lasting fruits on the female trees.

Holly, *Ilex* species. Holly shrubs and trees are dioecious, so only female hollies will make berries. Often these need a male pollinator somewhere near to set a good crop of red berries, but not always. Some female hollies will set a large crop of berries without any pollination at all. Fruit that sets without being pollinated is called *parthenocarpic fruit.*

Junipers, *Juniperus* species. Junipers, which are some of the most common landscape shrubs and trees in the world, are mostly separate sexed, but not all of them. When buying junipers, you only want female plants. You do not want junipers that have both sexes on the same plants (monoecious junipers), and you certainly don't want separate-sexed male junipers.

Of the many species of junipers that are dioecious (separate sexed), only the female plants will have the round, blue-green juniper berries. But all of the monoecious juniper species will have berries. In much of Utah, almost all the wild juniper trees are monoecious. They all have berries there. But in most other areas, only the female trees have fruit.

When buying junipers to plant, be sure to take a copy of *Allergy-Free Gardening* along with you and carefully compare the data. If you have a large juniper in your own yard, and it has fruit on it, that's a positive sign. But if you suspect it might be a monoecious species, you'll need to check and see if you can find the numerous small brown male pollen "cones" that are borne on the tips of the branches. If you're still confused on this one, pick a small branch of your juniper and take it to your county agriculture agent and see if he or she can identify it for you. If all else fails, email me and we'll get to the root of it eventually.

If you have allergies, one thing you don't need is a pollinating juniper in your own yard. A clear photo of a monoecious juniper is posted on my website, www.allergyfree-gardening.com.

Kaffir Plum trees, *Harpephyllum caffrum*. These trees, common in mild winter areas, only have the olive-sized red fruits on female trees. Males make nothing but pollen.

Kentucky Coffee Trees, *Gymnocladus dioica*. The female trees make big, dark seedpods. The male trees are much more popular because they don't make the big, messy seedpods, but they're the ones with the pollen.

Maple trees — female Red or Silver, *Acer* species; Box Elders; Devil's Maple; Horned Maple; and Ivy-Leafed Maple. In bloom, female maples will have small flowers that look a great deal like the winged seeds that they will eventually become. These seeds will always be paired in twos. This is also true for Box Elders, which are actually a type of maple tree. It is also true for some of the other separate-sexed maples such as Devil's Maple or Horned Maple, as well as the Ivy-Leafed Maple.

Mirror Plant, *Coprosma* species. This plant, of which there are many species, has small, soft, bright red berries on female plants only.

Mulberry trees, *Morus* species. Female mulberry trees produce large crops of messy fruits much favored by kids and birds (and this author). Male mulberry trees, sold as "fruitless" mulberry, produce huge amounts of very allergenic pollen. Weeping Mulberry is almost always a female form that has been top-grafted onto a seedling rootstock (or grafted onto a cutting-grown male mulberry).

Osage Orange trees, *Maclura pomifera*. These trees make baseball-sized, round orange fruits on the female trees only.

Oso Berry, *Oemleria cerasiformis*; and Silverberry, *Elaeagnus* species. These attractive, cold-hardy shrubs are all separate sexed and thus only form their small red or silver fruits on the female plants.

Palm trees and pepper trees, *Schinus* species. Female palm trees and female pepper trees will usually hang on to some fruit all year long. All pepper tree species and some species of palms are dioecious, separate sexed. If you have a pepper tree or, for example, a Phoenix Palm, Bismarck Palm, or Windmill Palm, and it has fruit on it, you're in luck. It's a female tree.

Pistache trees, *Pistacia* species. All pistache tree species are dioecious, and females will form clusters of small, often bright red fruits. Males produce none.

Podocarpus. *See yews and yew relatives.*

Poison ivy, *Rhus* species; and poison oak, *Toxicodendron* species. Both of these related species are separate sexed, and yes, pollen from the male plants can cause skin rash. You can actually get the rash without touching the plant. The pollen can come to you! Female poison oak or poison ivy plants form small, round, seethrough seeded fruits. Some birds actually eat these poison fruits, but don't touch them yourself!

Sassafras trees, *Sassafras albidum*. Sassafras trees produce small black fruits only if they're female. These trees will spread in the wild from roots that sprout. Sometimes an entire hillside will be covered with sassafras trees all of the same sex, essentially clones of each other. So if you have a male sassafras tree in your yard, be on the alert!

Shiny Xylosma; *Griselinia; Osmanthus;* and Laurel Snailseed, *Cocculus laurifolius*. With landscape shrubs such as Shiny Xylosma, *Griselinia, Osmanthus,* and Laurel Snailseed, the female plants may, if they're pollinated, form small, rounded black fruits.

Smoke Tree, *Cotinus* species; African Sumac; and Varnish Tree. The Smoke Tree and its other poison ivy–related relatives, like African Sumac and the Varnish Trees, only produce clusters of small, round, long-lasting, usually translucent watery fruits on the female plants.

Wax Myrtle, *Myrica* species. Wax Myrtle bushes only make clusters of the sweet-smelling, waxy berries if they're female.

Willows, *Salix* species, and poplar, *Populus* species. Willows and poplar are all dioecious. This includes all the cottonwoods, popples, and aspens. Their long, drooping flower clusters, called catkins, will have hundreds of tiny stamens, each tipped with a minute cluster of bright yellow pollen, if the tree is a male. Female flowers on willows and poplars look quite similar to the male flowers but lack the bright yellow-tipped stamens. So-called pussy willows are grown for their attractive flowers (catkins). These shrubs or small trees may be either male or female plants, but males are far more commonly used because they make the most attractive flowers.

Poplars or willows that produce "cotton," that fluffy material that blows all over the place in spring, are the female trees. The "cotton," often mistakenly blamed for causing allergies, is actually just masses of fluffy seeds.

Yews, *Taxus* species, and yew relatives (Yew Pines and Fern Pines), *Podocarpus* species. All yews and the yew relatives, Yew Pines and Fern Pines, are separate sexed. Female yews will set marble-sized, hard to miss, bright red fruits. Female *Podocarpus* make round, marble-sized, hard greenish-blue colored fruits that eventually turn a light yellow color. Males of all *Podocarpus* and yew species produce copious amounts of pollen that is both highly allergenic and quite poisonous.

With some of the less common separate-sexed shrubs such as the beautiful yewlike *Cephalotaxus* and the stiff-leafed evergreen *Torreya,* it is only the females that produce the grape-sized, round red fruits.

There are many other separate-sexed plants. Some are vines, houseplants, or cactuslike succulents. Others are trees or grasses. In all of these dioecious species only the females form seeds or fruits. With dioecious grasses, such as many of the **Bluegrass species** *(Poa)*, **Saltgrass** *(Distichlis spicata)*, or **Buffalo Grass** *(Buchloe dactyloides)*, it sometimes really does take an expert to tell the boys from the girls. But with most of the other species, you can usually do it yourself.

CHAPTER 4

Understanding OPALS

OPALS is the acronym for the Ogren Plant-Allergy Scale. I created this numerical scale some years ago to allergy-rank each plant listed in *Allergy-Free Gardening*. Many different factors went into the ranking process: How much pollen is produced, if any? How potent is this pollen? How much of the year is the plant in bloom? How big are the actual pollen grains? What is the *specific gravity* (density and weight) of each pollen grain? How sticky or dry are the grains? Is the tree perfect flowered, monoecious, dioecious, or polygamous? Does the sap cause dermatitis? Does the smell of the flowers bother people? These and other factors were weighted and compiled and became the foundation of the OPALS scale.

With OPALS, plants are ranked on a scale of 1 to 10. A plant ranked 1 is the least allergenic, and a plant ranked 10 is the most allergenic.

OPALS ranks each type of plant in relation to other plants of the same type. All perennials are ranked against other perennials. The shrubs are ranked according to other shrubs. And trees are ranked only against other trees.

A tree ranked 8 will have far more potential for allergy than will a perennial also ranked 8. This is simply because the tree is so much larger.

How to Use OPALS

Some people tell me they want to move to an area where the landscapes average 1 or 2 on the scale. "Good luck!" I tell them, for unfortunately there is no such place. The best thing people can do is to make their own places as allergy-free as possible. The next best thing to do is get involved at the city level and try to influence your own city council to enact a ban on the planting of any more highly allergenic trees in your neighborhood.

A plant with a ranking of 1 or 2 has very little potential for causing allergy. If the plant has a rank of 2 to 3, it still has very low potential to cause pollen allergy unless directly sniffed, but it may have potential to trigger skin rash from its sap.

Plants that rank from 1 to 5 should be considered low-risk plants. However, the allergy potential does rise as the number increases, so while there is little wrong with having a few 5s in the garden, you wouldn't want to plant too many of them.

Plants with allergy rankings of 10 are the worst. These can often cause both hay fever and asthma. They may also trigger skin rashes. A plant ranked 10 is known to cause the worst kind of allergy and to have the potential to affect a high number of people.

An Ideal Landscape

An ideal landscape will be high in diversity of plant materials. Diversity is important on many levels. Diversity often translates into fewer insect pests, molds, and other plant fungus diseases. An ideal landscape will have a number of female and other pollen-free plants. Any plants with high OPALS numbers will be placed far away from front or back doors, away from bedroom windows, away from patios and decks.

An ideal landscape will be well tended, and the plants in it will be especially well adapted to that particular area. Natives, if low in allergy potential, are quite useful, as are most low-pollen plants that will thrive in that particular region. Healthy plants are always a defense against allergy. Insect dander itself is highly allergenic, and pest insects produce honeydew on which mold thrives.

An ideal landscape is not dependent on chemical sprays but is one where disease-resistant plants are used.

An ideal landscape is home to many wild birds, and the soil beneath it is often home to an abundant supply of earthworms. Birds eat large numbers of insect pests, and earthworms aerate the soil and help keep the plants healthy.

An ideal landscape is a healthy place – a functional, pleasing place to just relax and enjoy. Stress aggravates all illnesses, and an ideal landscape is one that is stress reducing.

Factors Used to Build OPALS

More than a hundred possible factors are used to develop allergy rankings for plants. Each factor is either positive or negative. All factors are not weighted the same because some are more important than others. Most plants will have a combination of positive and negative factors that are computed to determine their OPALS ranking. If you already own a copy of *Allergy-Free Gardening* you can just check each plant for its OPALS number. But if you do not own the book, using the list of factors below, you can determine for yourself roughly how allergenic or nonallergenic a particular plant will be.

Following are some of the positive and negative factors used in building OPALS.

These are the things we want to find, factors that mean a plant has less potential to cause allergy.

- Perfect flowered. (The pollen doesn't need to travel far.)

- Large petals. (They attract pollinating insects, indicating less reliance on wind pollination. Anything that attracts pollinating insects is good, since pollen transported by insects, rather than the wind, is much less available to cause us allergies.)

- Brightly colored petals. (These also attract pollinating insects. Bright colors attract more insect pollinators than do pastel colors.)

- Flowers with nectar sources. (Nectar attracts pollinators.)

- Flowers where the male parts are deep inside the flower, as in a snapdragon. (The pollen is less exposed.)

- Polygamous with separate female flowers. (A plant like this has both perfect flowers and separate-sexed female flowers, and thus it has low pollen production and an excellent chance of attracting and trapping almost all of its own pollen.)

- A light pleasant scent. (It will draw pollinating insects.)

- Disease resistant. (It will have fewer pest insects and less disease, thus less insect dander and mold. Insect dander is not a problem associated with pollinating insects, such as honeybees. Dander is a definite problem, though, from plant-predatory, sucking pest insects such as mealybug, whitefly, scale, or aphids. Any botanical plant feature that limits pest insects is beneficial.)

- Female only. (Female plants have no pollen.)

- Pollen free but not strictly female. (Again, no pollen is always a plus.)

- Flowers colored red, orange, blue, or pink. (These colors attract the most pollinators, indicating little reliance on the wind.)

- Large-sized flowers. (Bigger flowers rely more on insect pollinators.)

- Very short bloom period. (Less time available for pollen production.)

- Blooms only on old wood. (The flowers, if allergenic, can be pruned away before they bloom.)

- Not in the same genus or family as any highly allergenic plants. (There is much less chance of interspecies cross-reactive allergic response. For example, if you are already allergic to poison oak, you will be at increased risk from its close relatives – pepper trees, mango, cashew, and sumac.)

- Sticky pollen. (It cannot travel easily in the air.)

- Pollen that is heavy, that has a high specific gravity. (Heavy pollen sinks faster, travels in air poorly.)

- In perfect-flowered plants, a ratio of one pistil to five stamens. (Fewer stamens mean less pollen per flower and also that a larger percentage of each flower's pollen may be trapped by that flower.)

- Brightly colored sepals. (It is another good indication of insect pollination. The sepals are underneath the petals, and colorful sepals will add to the attraction of the petals.)

- Monocarpic. (These plants only bloom once in their entire life cycle, and then they die, thus there is no pollen exposure until the plant's final year of life.)

- Does not bloom until very advanced in years. (Plants are pollen free for a longer period of time in the landscape.)

- Monoecious plants with abundant female flowers that are receptive to receiving pollen at the precise same time that male flowers of the same plant are releasing pollen. (A plant like this is designed by nature to trap its own pollen.)

- Monoecious plants with all the male flowers positioned above the female flowers. (A great example is the corn plant, where the tassels on the top have the pollen, and the ears of corn are collections of female flowers. The pollen is heavy, and gravity will bring it to the female flowers.)

There are other positive indicators, things that make a plant less likely to trigger allergies, but this ought to give you a good idea of what constitute positive factors.

SOME NEGATIVE FACTORS

These negative factors contribute to allergy-causing potential in any plant. The more of these factors any plant has, the worse its OPALS rank will be.

- Belongs to a family of plants well known to cause allergies. (Prime examples would be the Cashew, Olive, Spurge, and sunflower families. Here there is exceptional potential for interspecies cross-reactive allergenic responses.)

- May cause skin rash from contact with sap, flowers, or leaves. (This is self-explanatory.)

- Skin rash, when caused, is long lasting. (Certain plant-triggered cases of allergic dermatitis may persist for months.)

- Skin rash, when caused, is severe and may cause permanent scarring. (Sap from certain plants is not just allergenic, it is dangerous.)

- Very long bloom period. (Certain trees, like *Eucalyptus*, bloom for many months in the year, greatly increasing the pollen exposure around them.)

- Blooms on new wood, that is, wood grown in the current season. (Even if hard pruned, it will still bloom. The flowering is thus difficult to control by pruning or shearing.)

- Pollen grains light and dry, with low specific gravity. (This pollen will travel far and wide.)

- Pollen grains smaller than thirty microns. (Smaller pollen can be inhaled deeper, and it may also travel further in the wind.)

- Pollen grains completely round. (Round pollen travels well in the air.)

- Pollen grains with sharp spines. (This type of pollen can cause skin rash, dry skin, irritation of the nose, eyes, and throat. Sharp-spined pollen can also cause irritation simply from mechanical action rather than allergic response. Skin may be easily irritated by this itchy pollen, and when rubbed or scratched, it has a sandpaper effect resulting in rash or dry, flaky skin.)

- Pollen grains produced in large quantities. (This is never a plus with allergy control.)

- Pollen may cross-react with common food allergies. (Food allergies are on the rise, and cross-reactions with certain pollen types are common.)

- Male cultivar. (Cultivars are cloned plants, asexually propagated, and all male clones produce large amounts of pollen and trap none.)

- Strong fragrance known to trigger allergies. (Certain floral smells are well documented for provoking allergies.)

- Disagreeable odor from flowers or leaves. (Different odd plant odors can trigger allergic responses. These odors are actually composed of tiny allergenic airborne oils. You can't see them, but they are perfectly real.)

- Stamens exserted, that is, exposed. (These pollen-bearing stamens are more easily accessed directly or also from the movement of the air. They will be more likely to shed pollen.)

- In perfect-flowered plants, ratios of more than thirty stamens per stigma are negative. (Less pollen will be trapped per flower and more will be produced.)

- A polygamous plant with unisexual male flowers. (The male-only flowers will produce wind-borne pollen.)

- Light yellow, off-white, or greenish flowers. (Many of the most highly allergenic flowers are colored this way, which is unattractive to most pollinators.)

- Flowers lacking petals. (It is far less attractive to pollinators and more likely to have pollen that will move freely in the air.)

- Flowers lacking sepals. (Again, this usually means that a flower will be less attractive to insect pollinators.)

- Flowers are numerous and small. (This is the typical arrangement with most highly allergenic plants.)

- Monoecious flowered. (Production of unisexual male flowers usually is associated with airborne pollen.)

- Monoecious flowered with male flowers below the female flowers. (In monoecious plants this is an additional strong negative. A good example of this would be an Italian Cypress, where the female flowers are on the top of the plant and the male pollen flowers are on the bottom two-thirds. The cypress pollen must go *up* in order to pollinate. This system always involves large amounts of airborne pollen.)

- Pollen well known to cause asthma is strongly negative. (Pollen of some species, such as Castor Bean, frequently triggers serious bouts of asthma.)

- Lacks *nectaries* – the plant organs that hold the sugar-rich nectar. (No nectar makes the flowers less attractive to insect or animal pollinators and thus more reliant on the wind.)

- Has plant spores or sharp hairs that can cause skin, eye, bronchial, lung, or nasal mechanical irritation. (Certain plants, such as the sycamore tree, will have tiny, sharp material on their leaves or stems that can go airborne and cause allergy when inhaled. In some cases this will be more significant than their pollen.)

- Monoecious plants whose female flowers, relative to male flowers, are few in number. (Less pollen will be trapped and more will be in the air.)

- Monoecious plants whose female flowers are not receptive at the precise time that its male flowers release their pollen. (This plant, even though it produces female flowers, can trap none of its own pollen.)

- Non-native allergenic plants, known to spread quickly and to naturalize. (These domesticated plants can easily spread into wildlands and are then very difficult to eradicate. Landscape plants that naturalize cause a wide array of problems. They often upset the natural balance, forcing out native species of both plants and animals. Allergenic plants that may naturalize, such as *Casuarina,* are exceptionally troublesome.)

There are other factors used to allergy-rank plants, but this should give you a good idea of how it is done and what to look for.

Examples of OPALS

In each of the ten examples below, one particular plant or plant species is used to illustrate each degree of ranking. Reasons are given, positive or negative, or sometimes both, to explain how each ranking was determined. (A ranking of 1 is least allergenic, 10 is most allergenic.)

1. 'Autumn Glory,' Red Maple, *Acer rubrum* 'Autumn Glory' is a female tree. It traps pollen from male trees, produces no pollen itself, does not have spores or sharp hairs, has no sap or smell that causes allergies, is hardy, disease resistant, widely adapted, and in general doesn't cause allergies.

2. 'Golden Girl,' Chinese Maidenhair Tree, *Ginkgo biloba* 'Golden Girl' is always a female tree, has no pollen, traps pollen from male *Ginkgo* trees, and has numerous sticky flowers. The juice of the stinky fruits, however, can cause skin rash.

3. Pinks, carnations, *Dianthus* species, present very little opportunity for pollen allergy. They are not closely related to families of highly allergenic plants. They are insect pollinated, are both perfect flowered and complete flowered, have brightly colored petals, full sets of sepals, and have sticky pollen that is heavy and moderately large. But occasionally certain species, such as clove pinks, can trigger some allergy from their fragrance, and people who frequently handle *Dianthus* (usually carnations) as cut flowers sometimes get dermatitis from the sap.

4. Night-Blooming Jasmine, *Cestrum nocturnum*, has large, sticky pollen, is insect pollinated, has perfect flowers, has rich nectar sources, and is not known to cause skin rashes. But *Cestrum* also has a powerful fragrance that will often trigger allergies if it is planted too close to bedroom windows. The pollen, while not plentiful, is nonetheless poisonous. The flowers are also numerous and small. A substance that is poisonous

(toxic) will negatively affect everyone who ingests or inhales it. Pollen that is allergenic will usually only affect those with susceptible allergies.

5. Saint John's Wort, *Hypericum* species, is perfect flowered, has large, brightly colored petals, full sets of sepals, rich nectar sources, and is not in a family with numerous highly allergenic relatives. However, *Hypericum* has numerous male stamens, exserted (extended) stamens, produces considerable pollen, is pollinated by both wind and insects, and causes often fatal photodermatitis in animals that eat it.

6. The female Chinese Tallow Tree, *Sapium sebiferum,* is disease resistant where adapted, produces no pollen, and will trap pollen from male *Sapium* trees. The sap from the stems and leaves, however, has potential to be a strong allergen. The tree is in a family (Euphorbiaceae) well known to have many highly allergenic members, and the potential for cross-reactive allergy, especially to the sap, is considerable. People with allergy to latex have an even greater chance to react to *Sapium*. Male *Sapium* trees are ranked much worse, 10.

7. Shasta Daisy, *Chrysanthemum maximum,* has bisexual flowers, brightly colored petals, flowers of large size, is primarily pollinated by insects, and has sticky pollen. On the negative side, it belongs to a very highly allergenic family (Compositae), has numerous sharp-spined pollen grains, has a long bloom period, can cause skin rash, and has a disagreeable odor that can trigger allergies when it is used as a cut flower and brought inside the house. A few of these plants out in the yard represents little problem, but if brought inside they can be extremely allergenic.

8. Indian Stogie trees or Indian Cigar trees, *Catalpa,* are large flowered, brightly colored, have large petals, are perfect-flowered, are not known to cause skin rashes, are lightly scented,

and have rich nectar sources. On the negative side, though, they are too commonly used, they are *amphipilous* (pollinated by both wind and insects), and their pollen is well known to cause allergies. *Catalpa* stamens are numerous and exserted, and as legumes that shed pollen, they may present special difficulties with cross-reactivity for children with existing dangerous allergies to peanuts.

9. Primrose Tree, *Lagunaria patersonii,* is perfect flowered, insect pollinated, has nectar sources and large, brightly colored flowers. Negatives of this tree are that it has many stamens, all of them exserted (extended from the flowers), and the flowers are numerous. The bloom period is quite long, and the tree produces extremely large numbers of minute, needle-sharp stinging hairs that can cause asthma if inhaled, skin rash, and severe irritation to the eyes when contacted. Almost all of the hazards from this tree will be highly localized, confined to the immediate area surrounding the tree.

10. 'Shamel,' California Pepper Tree, *Schinus molle* 'Shamel,' is a male cultivar (clone) developed because it is seedless and thus "litter-free." 'Shamel' produces large amounts of highly allergenic pollen every year, blooming for a long period of time. Although insects often visit it, it also produces airborne pollen. The flowers are tiny, pale yellow, extremely numerous, and are all imperfect and male. The odor of the flowers is odd, attracts flies, and may cause allergy for some. The sap from these trees can cause persistent, delayed-reaction skin rash that is very similar to poison ivy or poison oak rash. Crushed leaves from this tree produce volatile oils that can trigger allergies. Fumes from the wood can cause allergy if it is burned.

   The 'Shamel' pepper tree is large and blooms profusely at an early age. Allergies to the pollen and odors of this tree and all members of the *Schinus* family are well documented and common. The trees, which are widely used, are in the Cashew family, known to contain some of the most highly allergenic trees, shrubs, and vines in the world. *Schinus* may cross-react with any of its relatives, such as Varnish Tree, mango, poison oak, Poison Sumac, or poison ivy.

Trade Secrets

Why, I've been asked, am I giving away the secrets to determining OPALS rankings? For many years there has been a real need for a system such as this. I am not giving away all the secrets here, but I am sharing many of them. This leaves my work wide open to copycats, and I understand that. I choose to share this information because there are plenty of skeptics out there. They have asked, rightfully so, "How did he ever come up with such a ranking system? What is it based on?"

Well, here are the answers to those questions. OPALS is based on the above factors, and on other similar negative or positive botanically, horticulturally, or medically related indicators.

CHAPTER 5

Avoiding Allergies with the Right Native Plants

M any of our most allergenic plants commonly used in land-scaping in the United States and Canada are indeed native to North America. However, it is the gender manipulation of these plants by commercial horticulture that has caused most of the huge increases we are now experiencing with allergy problems.

American Elms

The number one street tree in America for many years was the tall, stately American Elm, *Ulmus americana*. The American Elm used to grace the streets of thousands of towns and cities, but when Dutch Elm disease (DED) started to spread and kill off these na-tive elms in the 1960s, the insect-pollinated, perfect-flowered elms were most often replaced with wind-pollinated, unisexual-flowered street trees. Most often used were dioecious male ash, poplars, and maples, and monoecious trees, especially oaks and sycamores. Almost all the replacement trees were native, and males clones were preferred since they were "litter-free."

Many things happened because of the big switch from the elms to these other tree species. In addition to allergy increases, there were other negative environmental consequences from this overuse of male clones. The elm flowers were a rich nectar source, and since elm trees bloomed very early in the season, at a time when other insect food sources were severely limited, urban honeybees and butterflies depended on this food source.

Since the majority of the street trees used to replace the elms were wind-pollinated, they often lacked these nectaries and supplied no early-season food source. Soon we started to see a rapid decline in the total numbers of urban honeybees and butterflies. There were other factors as well behind this decline – pollution, insecticides, and disease – but the loss of the crucial early-season food sources should not be underestimated.

DED spread mostly from east to west across the United States and so has the rise in allergy rates. One can actually track the spread of allergy in the United States from the decline of the elms. DED started first in the eastern United States and then slowly spread westward, killing off all the elms as it spread. The areas that were hit first were the first to plant replacement trees. These same areas were also the first to experience the explosion of pollen-allergy cases as soon as the new trees grew large enough to flower and produce pollen. Eventually DED reached cities on the Pacific Coast and killed off their elms. Fifteen years later, with the wind-pollinated replacement trees planted and blooming, allergy rates in the West finally caught up with the East.

The urban landscape before Dutch Elm disease struck was, of course, a highly manipulated environment itself, but the trees were seedlings, not asexually propagated clones. (A seedling tree is a tree that was grown from seed rather than having been budded or grafted. A seedling tree is not a cultivar – it is not a clone.)

Manipulation of the green environment is something we do all the time in horticulture. The old elm tree–lined streets were hardly good examples of environmental soundness, but at least they had sexual balance.

The American Elms did cause a certain amount of low-level, early spring allergy, simply because they were so very common. The overplanting of elms resulted in a lack of biodiversity and set the stage for the massive kill from DED. We now know that it is always a mistake to use a monoculture, that is, to overplant one species. Too much of one thing eventually results in excessive insect pests and disease. Diversity is always a good idea in horticulture.

Diversity

Nature itself is always highly diverse, and biodiversity is the way to go when we are creating landscapes that will limit allergenic exposure. Almost any species of plants can eventually cause allergies if it is overplanted. All too often in our contemporary urban landscapes, we see that landscapers have used the same old plants again and again. This simplistic approach results in landscapes that lack originality and produce a numbing "sameness" in much of our urbanscape. When residential houses are professionally landscaped with the exact same plant materials used to landscape banks, real estate offices, and mortuaries, we all lose.

Pollen allergies today are far worse in cities than in the country, despite the fact that there is much more total green matter in the countryside than in the city. Plant selection has been the main problem.

Natives and Urban Male Landscapes

Many different native trees and shrubs are used in our landscapes. Maples, oaks, locust, poplars, willows, catalpa, birch, junipers, and many others are used extensively. Unfortunately in each regional area only a few species are typically used. But our urbanscapes not only require a diversity of species; they also require a diversity of sex. Unfortunately the plant breeders and propagators discovered how to "sex-out" the trees and shrubs. They learned to use only male plants, ironically as "mother plants," as the source for their scion wood for asexual propagation. First they just used male plants from the dioecious (separate-sexed) species, but later they learned how to produce all-male clones from species that in nature were never unisexual (the monoecious species).

For example, Honey Locust trees, *Gleditsia triacanthos,* are native to the southeastern United States. Look at these trees in the wild and you will see that all of them are almost always covered with long seedpods. But go to a nursery now and look at the Honey Locust trees for sale. Inevitably they are called "seedless" – they are in effect all-male clones. With Honey Locust and many other monoecious species, one branch may have only male flowers and another only female. The propagators took their scion material (wood for grafting, budding, or cuttings) only from the male branches, and the results became male trees.

What exactly is the effect of using all-male cloned trees and shrubs in our landscapes? Very simply, this translates to an excess of allergenic pollen.

Unhealthy Trees Create Mold Spores

Much of our allergy problem is caused by tiny airborne reproductive mold spores. These spores are usually much smaller even than pollen grains, and like pollen they may be potent allergens.

Plants (trees especially) that are not healthy will almost always be attacked by pests, especially by aphids, scale, mealybugs, and whiteflies. These insects suck the vital plant juices, weakening the tree further. Feces secreted by these insects are commonly called "honeydew," and this honeydew is very nutrient rich. Almost immediately mold will grow on this fertile substance, and quickly the mold will start to reproduce itself with its billions of tiny spores.

If you look up at a tree and the leaves look dirty, this is almost always because they are indeed filthy and are covered with insects and mold. Often a tree like this will produce incredible amounts of mold spores for many months on end. In a mild southern climate, this mold formation can go on year round. Essentially, having a tree like this on your property is much like having a giant puffball mushroom in your yard. The mushroom continually showers everyone nearby with allergenic spores. (Mushrooms are a type of fungus. They reproduce by their millions of spores, which are also quite allergenic.) Sometimes, especially on extremely high traffic streets, a tree's leaves simply are dirty – or rather, covered in black soot. These trees will almost always fail to thrive so will eventually attract insects and as a result begin to shed mold spores.

Why Are These Trees Sickly?

There are many reasons why a tree fails to thrive. The insects on the tree are not really the cause; they're just a reflection of a more fundamental problem. Usually a tree is unhealthy because it is not the best tree for that particular spot. This is where natives play such an important role. A tree that is native to an area will be much more likely to thrive there.

In the July/August 2000 issue of *Wild Ones Journal,* there was an excellent article by Andy Wasowski entitled "Provenance," in which he explored the concept that being truly native means being endemic to one particular area. For example, just because Black Ash *(Fraxinus nigra)* is native to the United States does not mean that it would thrive in Southern California. Black Ash is endemic to areas of the United States where the winters are cold and long, the soil is acidic, and the water table is high. Black Ash will thrive in a cold, damp landscape in northern Minnesota, but it will not do well in hot, dry, alkaline Los Angeles.

The problem, though, is that a Black Ash, because it is inherently a tough, sturdy tree, might grow if planted in a place like Los Angeles. It might even grow to become a fairly large tree, but it would never be a very healthy one. And thus, this tree – out of place, not in an area very similar to where it originated – will almost certainly become a mold spore factory, an allergy tree.

We who love horticulture often want to grow plants that are not well suited to our areas. We are forever planting trees that we like in areas where they will not thrive. Rarely do we think it all out, years into the future, and consider the unhealthy ramifications of this process.

Corruption of the Natives

This whole business of tidy landscapes has gotten out of control. Our desire to manipulate nature is starting to backfire on us. The all too common practice of using natives and asexually manipulating their sexes for the purpose of low-maintenance plantings is quickly becoming a very unhealthy situation.

Here is a true story I've told many times.

I was out in a neighborhood near mine in San Luis Obispo, California. I had my camera in hand and needed some close-up photos of male Coyote Brush *(Baccharis pilularis)*. I was standing on the public sidewalk taking shots with my macro lens when an older fellow walked out of the house. He stared at me and then asked, "What in the world could be worth photographing in my front yard?"

I explained that I am an allergy researcher and I needed photos of male Coyote Brush in bloom.

"Something wrong with them?" he asked me.

"They're all male," I said, "and they are closely related to ragweed. Your whole front yard is covered with this stuff."

"Hmm," he said, frowning.

"Actually, sir," I said, "all your ground cover is male. That entire row of junipers there on the side of your house, they're all males too. Notice that none of them have any juniper berries?"

"Uh, huh," he said.

"This ash tree in your yard – there are no seeds on it either. Ash always makes seeds if it's a female tree, but this one is a male too. They're an olive relative and the pollen of the males is quite allergenic." I looked over his entire landscape. "Actually," I said, "everything in your yard is highly allergenic, everything except for that climbing rosebush on your porch."

"Figures," he said.

"So," I asked, "does anyone here have allergies?"

"Sure," he told me, "my wife does. She's got terrible allergies."

"I'd be willing to bet she's having them right now," I said.

"Yep," he said, " she's been sick for several weeks now."

Now, when I think of that particular landscape, the use of manipulated natives is quite interesting. The groundsel bush ground cover is native to California, and endemic to the coastal region where San Luis Obispo is located. The juniper growing alongside the house is also a thriving native species, and even the large ash tree in the yard is a California native. But the ground cover had all been grown from cuttings of dioecious male plants. The ash tree, originally a seedling, had been grafted or budded with scion wood from a "seedless" male tree. The junipers had also all been originally propagated by cuttings, using only wood from male plants. In the above case the landscape was high in natives, but it was not in the least bit natural.

Natural Resource Management

Recently I have started to think of my work as a form of natural resource management (NRM). I am trying to get us back to landscapes that are natural, that are diverse, that use plants that will thrive, that use a blend of plants that are sexually balanced. In nature we never find landscapes composed of just one sex; there is a sexual equilibrium.

The resource we are managing is the very air we breathe. Excessive pollen or mold spores are pollutants, biopollutants perhaps, but toxic, allergenic, asthma-causing, respiratory-clogging pollutants nonetheless. Clean fresh air is priceless.

For too long now our urban landscapes have been managed with little or no regard to their effect on the health of the people living in these landscapes. It is time now to start actively managing our landscapes. Now is the time to take control and to get back to a more natural state.

CHAPTER 6

Low-Allergy and Allergy-Free Ground Covers

A good ground cover is one that stays low, establishes quickly, is largely insect and disease free, and does not produce a lot of pollen. I am frequently asked to recommend low-allergy ground covers, as many people today want to switch from growing and mowing lawns to planting ground covers. Here are some useful ground cover plants to consider. There are many others just as good, but these are among the easiest to find in nurseries.

In zones 3–10, *Ajuga repens,* or **Carpet Bugle,** is often useful as a low-allergy ground cover for smaller areas. It is much easier to establish where summer rains are common. In some southern states, it does escape into the woods and naturalize. (Domestic plants that establish themselves in the wild are said to "naturalize.") In the drier West, it will grow all right but only if watered regularly. *Ajuga* will grow in sun or shade but often does best in shady or semi-shady spots. *Ajuga* is low growing, has small blue flowers, and attractive, dark, bronzy-green leaves.

In mild winter areas (zones 9–10), ***Aptenia cordifolia,*** or **Red Apple Iceplant,** is very low allergy and grows easily and fast. Red Apple spreads quickly and can be planted from unrooted cuttings. It will grow in full sun or in the shade. Once it is established it is quite drought tolerant. Red Apple is good for steep hillsides, and it is very nonflammable, which is also a plus. Bees love the bright little red flowers. Red Apple will stay lower in full sun than it will in the shade.

Arctostaphylos, or **manzanita,** has much going for it. Manzanita is low allergy, drought tolerant, and longer lived than many other ground covers. There are many different manzanita species used for ground covers, and they vary greatly in winter hardiness. The most winter hardy of all of them, ***Arctostaphylos uva-ursi,*** or **Bearberry,** will grow in all zones. Manzanita as ground cover appears to be gaining in popularity, and this is a trend certainly to be encouraged.

Winter hardy in zones 3–10, ***Buchloe dactyloides,*** or **Buffalo Grass,** can make a good allergy-free ground cover if a female cultivar is used. As of this writing, the best cultivar is one called 'Legacy.' 'Legacy' is blue-green in color, stays very low, often well under six inches tall, and is very drought tolerant once established. 'Legacy' grows best in full sun but tolerates shade better than the older types of Buffalo Grass. 'Legacy' can also be used as a no-mow ground cover for hillsides.

The main drawback to all kinds of Buffalo Grass is that they are summer grasses and turn completely dormant in winter. This makes them less useful in zone 10. However, they can be mowed short and overseeded with winter annual grasses if needed. Also, in my own tests I have found that occasionally 'Legacy' will throw up some male pollen-bearing flower heads. This pollen is sterile but, nonetheless, not desired by any means. When I mowed the 'Legacy' once a month, it never produced any pollen flowers. I have also been testing a female clone called '609,' and it has never produced any male flowers.

'Legacy,' '609,' or other female Buffalo Grass clones can be bought either as plugs or as sod. It takes about a season to fill in totally when planted from plugs planted six inches apart. Buffalo Grass grown from seed will contain many male plants and is not recommended.

Carissa grandiflora, or **Natal Plum,** is another good, low growing, attractive, shrubby ground cover for mild winter areas. In zones 8–10, it is easy to grow, long lasting, and very low allergy. Natal Plum leaves are shiny green, the flowers are bright white, and the fruits are cherry red. It does, however, have sharp thorns. Certain cultivars stay lower than others.

Dichondra makes a nice, very low-growing, low-allergy ground cover or lawn substitute for zones 8–10. It does take regular watering, weeding, and fertilizing, though, to maintain it. *Dichondra* will grow in sun or shade but will be much lower in full sun. *Dichondra* would be better for smaller areas and is not suitable as a ground cover for hillsides or any large areas. It is not as tough as a grass sod, but you can walk on it. *Dichondra* produces very little pollen, and when grown right, it is extremely attractive. *Dichondra* can be grown from seed or planted from flats.

The *Juniperus* **species** include some very useful, low-growing, pollen-free female cultivars. Some species are hardy in almost all zones. 'Bar Harbor,' 'Glenmore,' and 'Icee Blue' are three very low-growing, pollen-free female cultivars of *Juniperus* that are useful in zones 3–10.

In zones 7–10, *Vinca major,* the larger and faster-growing form of the perennial **Periwinkle,** makes a very good low-allergy ground cover, and it is one that is suitable for large areas and hillsides.

Occasionally people get skin rash from the sap of these plants, but this is not common. *Vinca major* grows fast and will grow in full sun or in deep shade. It has nice blue flowers, dark green leaves, and much to recommend it. As a ground cover for a large area, it is certainly better than other more common plants such as honeysuckle, ivy, and acacia.

In zones 3–7, **Vinca minor** can make a very fine, low, long-lasting, low-allergy ground cover. It is not very fast growing, but if kept well watered, weeded, and fertilized, it grows steadily. *Vinca minor*, also called **Periwinkle,** has blue flowers and is long lived. Note that *Vinca minor* is much more winter hardy than is *Vinca major*. Also, much annual *Vinca* is sold, often as *Vinca rosea* or as *Catharanthus roseus*. While this is a fine plant for warm, sunny areas, it is not winter hardy and is unsuitable as a ground cover.

CHAPTER 7

Houseplants and Indoor Air Quality

We have been discussing only outdoor plants up to this point, but what about the plants we grow inside the house? Houseplants can be the source of cleaner air, but they can also be the source of allergies.

In general, houseplants that are exceptionally healthy will be the healthiest plants to keep in our homes. Insect pests on houseplants and the related health problems caused by them are always a concern. But so too are certain houseplants that may shed pollen or ones that are known to release other harmful substances into the air. In this chapter, we'll explore those houseplants that are the best choices for our homes, and how to maintain them so that we have the cleanest possible indoor air.

Insects?

Yes, greenhouse insect pests are now extremely resistant to all kinds of insecticides. As a result, many healthy looking houseplants we buy are often already infested with bugs. Always look over a new houseplant carefully before buying it. Be sure to look under the leaves, too, for signs of whitefly. Whiteflies are tiny, and they are bright white. They will usually be on the underside of leaves and will fly off if touched. It is now difficult in many areas to be able to buy, for example, any poinsettias that are not already infested with whitefly.

In addition, any houseplants that do not thrive will eventually get infested with insects, especially mealybugs, aphids, whiteflies, scale, or spider mites. All of these insects can quickly explode in numbers and can present a serious allergy problem. Insects shed old skin and other body parts, and this insect dander is very allergenic.

Where do these insects come from, and how do they get on our houseplants in the first place? Good questions. Some insect pests may simply fly through the front door when it's open, and other ones will hatch from minute larvae that are living in the potting soil. But for the most part the plants are already infested when you buy them, and when conditions are right, out they come.

As previously mentioned, sucking insects, such as scale, mealybugs, aphids, and whiteflies, produce large amounts of feces called "honeydew," and on this rich organic material mold quickly grows. The mold then produces reproductive mold spores, and these spores become airborne inside the house. Mold spores are, of course, quite allergenic.

The answer to insects is to keep the plants healthy. First, we should only use houseplants that are well adapted to growing inside the house. They should get the kind of light they need or they will get buggy. Spider mites thrive in hot weather. Whiteflies flourish in cool weather. Houseplants should be kept well fertilized. Lack of fertilizer will eventually result in a plant that is weak and that will then be attacked by insect pests. I like time-release fertilizers for all houseplants because they rarely burn the plants and they keep working for months.

Time-release fertilizers come in three-month and nine-month formulations. I add a teaspoon of time-release fertilizer to each four-inch pot, placing it right on top of the soil. Larger pots get more. Think of this as fertilizer insurance. In addition to time-release fertilizers, I also like to use water-soluble fertilizers at least once a month, more often in summer and less often in winter. For most water-soluble fertilizers, a teaspoon to a gallon of water is about right.

It is always a good idea to let houseplants dry out a little bit between watering. This gives the roots a chance to get more air and also discourages the growth of molds in the soil. When you do water houseplants, it is wise to soak them thoroughly rather than give them just a little bit of water each time. Always use water that is lukewarm, at least at room temperature. Most houseplants are tropicals and they do not tolerate cold roots well. (If you have a ceramic water-catching saucer underneath the pot and this saucer holds water for long periods of time, you may well be drowning the roots of the plant. Remove the saucer and dump it. Remember, roots need air!) Some people have very good luck by placing their houseplant pots in large dishpans with an inch of so of water and letting the plants wick the water up from the bottom. Once the soil in the pots is all moist, they're removed from the pan. This method is time-consuming, but it is effective.

At least once a year all houseplants should be flushed with plain water to remove salt buildup. To do this, simply soak the container from the top until water pours out of the bottom. Wait a few minutes and repeat the heavy soaking. This will help leach the salt out of the pot.

If the tips of the leaves on your houseplants consistently die or look burned, your household tap water may contain too much fluoride for good growth. Another situation that will ruin house-plants is water that has been through a "water softener." These machines use rock salt, and the resulting water is often too salty for good plant growth. If either of the above are problems, I suggest that as often as possible you water with rainwater or with bottled spring water.

Houseplants should be kept clean too. Often dust will stick on the leaves, and unless they are washed clean on a regular basis, houseplants can be regular dust piles. The dust on the leaves clogs up the plant's pores and also cuts down on its ability to photosynthesize. Dust is, of course, an allergen. Wipe down the leaves of houseplants with some clean water and a sponge. Add a tiny bit of dish soap to the water when you wipe them down, a teaspoon to a gallon. Use lukewarm water. The soap will help make the leaves cleaner, and it will kill some insects.

If you find insects on a houseplant, take it outside, put it in the shade, and spray it thoroughly with a mix of dish soap and vegetable oil. Use several tablespoons of each to a gallon of warm water. Spray the plants every day for a week. If this doesn't get rid of the bugs, then consider dumping them. If the plants are valuable or you just can't bear to part with them, add some neem oil to the above insecticide mix and spray them with this several more times. Neem is a natural insecticide made from the Indian neem tree. Neem is safe, effective, and besides killing insects, it has some fungicidal qualities as well. Neem is now marketed by a number of different companies.

Scale are insect pests that form colonies on the stems and under the leaves of plants. They usually look like small brown scales, hence their name. Scale is not easy to get rid of. Sometimes to kill scale on a houseplant I will pour some vegetable oil in a cup and then just brush it directly on the scale with a small paintbrush. In very few cases does the oil ever damage the leaves of the plants, and it will smother the scale. This also will work with mealybugs.

Do not bring buggy plants back into the house! Even after you get rid of the pests on the plant, before you return it to your house you need to ask why it got buggy in the first place. Is the light too weak? Is the air in the house too dry? Have you been neglecting to feed it enough? Has it been kept too dry? Too wet? Is it too cold inside? Too hot? Whatever the answer, you'll need to change something in order to get it to thrive.

Make a habit of looking over the leaves and stems of all your houseplants on a regular basis. Look on the stems for scale. Look under the leaves for other insect or mite pests. Spider mites are tiny, reddish in color, and look like miniature spiders. They also may form webs on the undersides of leaves. One of the best ways to control spider mites is to wash down the plants frequently.

Dander from spider mites is especially allergenic, and any plant that continues to get infested with mites ought to be tossed. One last tip here: In areas where the fall and spring months are cool, you can place a spider mite–infested plant outside for a few hours in weather that is cold but above freezing; 35 to 45 degrees will work fine. This blast of cold will kill the spider mites but not the plant. Just don't leave it out overnight that time of year, since no houseplants tolerate frost or freezing weather.

Keep your houseplants bug-free and they'll add to your healthy home.

VOCs and Houseplants?

All plants release a certain amount of "biogenic emissions" into the air. The emissions are polluting volatile organic compounds (VOCs), and they are a valid cause for concern. Some plants release only a small amount and then consume much more than they release. The ones to worry about are the plants that release more than they consume. Chief among the plant-produced VOC pollutants are carbon monoxide and ozone. Both of these are primary elements of smog. Smog has been shown to aggravate existing allergies and to cause allergies itself. Other VOC gases of allergy concern inside houses (but not necessarily produced by plants) are formaldehyde, benzene, xylene, toluene, ammonia, acetone, methyl alcohol, ethyl acetate, and trichlorethylene.

Ficus trees release almost no airborne pollen. Unfortunately Ficus, and especially the common houseplant tree Ficus benjamina, are high emitters of VOCs. Does this mean we should not plant Ficus trees? Yes and no. Yes, an occasional Ficus tree in the yard here and there poses very little problem, but lining entire streets with Ficus trees is not a good plan. Ficus benjamina as a houseplant? Not a great idea if you have allergies.

At any rate, Ficus often fail to thrive in houses since most household light is too weak for them and most household air is too dry. They will often be infested with spider mites or other insects, and these will just add to the VOC problem. VOCs are not good for people with allergies. Actually, VOCs are not good for anyone.

Which Houseplants Are VOC Consumers?

Some years ago NASA scientists discovered that certain plants can remove considerable amounts of VOCs from the air. The plants listed below are said to be quite effective at removing indoor pollutants. Please keep in mind, though, that they must be healthy, and they must be kept bug free in order to work.

Arrowhead Vine, *Syngonium podophyllum*

Chinese Evergreen, *Aglaonema modestrum*

Dendrobium species, orchids

Dracaena, *Dracaena marginata*

Dumb Cane, *Dieffenbachia* species

Dwarf banana plants, *Musa* species

Golden Pothos, *Pothos aureus*

Moth Orchid, *Phalaenopsis* species

Norfolk Island Pine, *Araucaria heterophylla*

Red Emerald Philodendron, *Philodendron domesticum*

Schefflera, *Schefflera* species

Snake Plant, *Sansevieria trifasciata*

Spider Plant, *Chlorophytum comosum*

Wax Begonia, *Begonia* species

Also said to be good for cleaning indoor air are *Rhapis, Chamaedorea,* and Phoenix Palms, but it is important to note here that only female palms should be used. You don't need palm pollen in your house.

CHAPTER 8

Eliminating Molds and Allergy-Causing Mold Spores

Both indoors and out, molds and the spores they produce are harmful to plants and to humans nearby. Because it is so important and so often overlooked, bear with me as I repeat a message here and elsewhere in this book. All plants that are grown under poor conditions (too little light, too much water, etc.) will get infested with insects, which will secrete "honeydew." On this very nutrient-rich, gooey substance, mold grows quickly. The molds then start producing spores, and soon there is a serious allergy situation.

Mold spores have proteins that are especially allergenic. They are tiny, usually much smaller than individual pollen grains. Because they are so small, they can be inhaled deeper, which adds to their potential for causing problems. In addition, when mold grows all over the leaves of plants, it coats the leaves of the plants, robbing them of needed sunshine and further weakening the plant.

Fortunately there are many things we can do in our gardens and landscaping to eliminate molds and their allergy-causing spores.

How to Keep Your Plants Mold Free

Let's explore the numerous things we can do to get rid of mold in our yards. Mold inside of houses and apartments has been recognized in the past few years as a serious problem, but what few people realize is that high levels of mold spores from the surrounding landscape are actually much more common. Keep in mind that mold spores can easily pass right through the tightest window screen.

LOCATION, LOCATION, LOCATION

Whether we have mold in our houses and in our yards may depend on what we plant and where we plant it. If there is a rule number one, it is: do not plant evergreen trees on the south side of your house!

I continually see evergreen trees or shrubs, which will eventually get tall, being planted on the south side of the house. In the winter when the sun is low on the horizon, we get most of our light and warmth from the sunlight that shines from the south. On cold winter mornings our warm early morning light comes from the east, and it is never a good idea to block that with tall evergreens.

A house with tall evergreen trees on the south, east, or southeast corners is one that will always be cold and damp in the winter months. And cold and damp are exactly what mold thrives on.

The best place for tall evergreens is on the north side of our houses. There they will not block any needed winter light and warmth, but they will act as a windbreak and provide protection from cold north winds.

Deciduous trees are perfect for planting on the south and east sides of homes. In the hot summer months deciduous trees will be all leafed out and will keep the house behind them nice and cool. In the cold winter months they will be bare of leaves, and the low sunlight will shine through and warm things up. In this day and age of exploding energy costs, it is just downright silly to plant evergreens where they don't belong. For stopping mold spores, using deciduous trees on the southeastern exposures is the only way to go.

CHOOSE YOUR MULCHES CAREFULLY

Many people seem unclear on just exactly what mulch is. Very simply, mulch is anything that covers the soil. Mulch holds down weeds and cuts down on summer water loss. Earthworms often thrive under mulch, and in general mulches usually help plants grow better. Mulches can be made of old leaves, straw, rocks, bark, gravel, boards, bricks, or even plastic.

Mulches are almost always a very good idea, but when it comes to fighting off molds, mulches aren't all created equally. The trouble with bark is that it can get moldy. Don't use bark mulches in areas where there is a lot of moisture. Gravel, stone, and brick mulches are good because they don't encourage mold growth. I like smooth gravels, river gravel, which is easy on bare feet. Flat stones or cement pavers make decent mulches, are easy on the feet, and in the right spot, they look good as well.

In many areas you can now get free mulch, which is made up mostly of chipped trees and shrubs, from the city or county. In the West there is much free *Eucalyptus* mulch to be had, but it isn't very good, since few things grow well in it because of its oiliness. The same can be said for mulch chips made from walnut trees. Neither *Eucalyptus* nor walnut mulch is worth the trouble of spreading it. Newspaper mulches, by the way, not only look trashy, but they also grow lots of mold.

The one spot where even the best mulches are less effective is in those cold, always shaded areas. Here mulch will keep the soil from ever warming up. Everywhere else though, the right type of mulch is useful.

CHOOSE YOUR PLANTS CAREFULLY

If a tree is native to the cold, damp forests of Japan or Minnesota, it just won't thrive in a place like Los Angeles. It might grow in Los Angeles, though, and that's the problem: it will grow there, but it won't thrive. Because it doesn't have the conditions it needs, it will always be weak, and pests always prey on the weak. Remember, insect pests equal mold spores.

Judicious use of natives is often one of the very best ways to avoid many of these weak plants–mold problems. However, make sure the "natives" you buy are endemic to your own particular area. Also, make sure you're not getting a bunch of male (pollen-producing) clones. Many of the native trees, shrubs, and ground covers sold now are male clones.

TREAT YOUR PLANTS WELL

There are many things we can do to keep our plants healthy. Landscape plants thrive only when we supply them with what they need. These needs will vary widely from one species to another.

Give Your Plants Room to Breathe and Bask in the Sunlight

Since mold grows best in cool, dark, damp places, bright light and fresh air are the enemies of mold. In every location there are prevailing winds, that is, the breeze blows primarily from one direction. Many landscapes are so plugged up and crowded that the breeze simply can't penetrate the mess. A landscape with no airflow is one where molds will thrive. Molds grow best in conditions with poor air circulation.

If your own yard is overgrown and choked for lack of fresh air, then get out the pruning saw and start thinning it out. Clean, fresh air, free to move about, equals less mold and fewer mold spores.

You may also need to prune overhead branches that are blocking sunlight. Consider hiring a tree trimmer to thin out some of the branches overhead. Open the trees up so that the sunlight can come through. Perhaps it would be a good idea to actually remove a tree or two if they're growing too close. Let the light shine!

When planting any new tree, consider the shade that it will cast when it is full-grown. Certain trees always develop very thick canopies while others will be light and airy.

Just Enough Water

Perhaps as important as any other single mold factor is the watering. Too little water makes weak plants that attract insects. Too much water will also always produce weak plants. Each type of plant has its own water requirements, and these may differ widely from species to species. It is always a wise idea in the landscape to group plants according to their water requirements. Keep the drought-tolerant ones in one area and the thirsty ones in another. This makes it much simpler to irrigate accordingly.

Automatic irrigation systems with timers are responsible for a great deal of mold growth. Allergists in desert areas like Las Vegas and Tucson often find very high mold spore counts in the middle of the summer! Much of this is directly caused by irrigation systems that are not being monitored closely enough. Often they are set to irrigate lawns that are already still soggy from the last watering. Overwatered lawns will quickly become mold factories and will shower everyone near them with an abundance of mold spores.

Watch out too for sprinklers that soak the foundations of the house. Indoor mold is often caused by outdoor watering mistakes.

Plant Diseases and Spores

Many plant pests are not insects or molds but are fungal-type diseases such as mildew, rust, black spot, scab, and leaf blight. These organisms all produce allergenic airborne spores. The very best way to avoid these diseases and their spores is by planting disease-resistant plants. To find the most resistant plants, read plant tags and research trees or shrubs before you buy them. Then, keep plants growing cleanly and strongly, following the same guidelines as outlined for mold reduction. Insect-attacked plants will often later be attacked by fungus diseases, and vice versa. Healthy plants go a long way to keeping our air clean.

Certain plants if grown in the wrong area can almost be counted on to harbor disease.

- Evergreen *Viburnum* growing in the shade will certainly get moldy and full of mildew.

- Crape Myrtle trees grown in an area that doesn't have hot summers will always have mildew.

- A cold, wet spring frequently brings out a huge flush of both mildew and the fungus *anthracnose* on the leaves of California sycamore trees.

- In areas with cool, foggy nights and warm days, rust will surely grow on any roses, hollyhocks, or snapdragons that are not rust resistant.

- Most roses grown in too much shade will quickly mildew. Actually, almost any plant that thrives in full sun will run into problems in too much shade.

Insecticides and Fungicides

When you see a plant covered with insects or fungus, fight the immediate urge to go get out the chemical sprays. Many chemical sprays will themselves trigger allergies. They may also weaken your immune system.

A shrub full of insects can often be helped immensely by just blasting off the bugs with a strong jet of water from the garden hose. Spider mites can also often be brought under control with this same stiff spray of water.

Many insect pests can be killed with a simple, nontoxic homemade spray of vegetable oil, water, and liquid dish-washing soap. For a gallon of water add two tablespoons of vegetable oil and two to four tablespoons of soap. I like Ivory Liquid but have used other brands with good success. If the insects are not controlled with this mix, make it stronger. I sometimes use a mix with as much as ten tablespoons of soap and ten of oil. Some plants tolerate this mix better than others. Experiment and remember that it is always safer (for the plants) to spray early in the day rather than in the heat of the day.

For fungus diseases spray them with a mix of baking soda, dish soap, and water. Baking soda is a natural fungicide. Depending on how bad the infestation of disease is, I use from two to six tablespoons of baking soda per gallon of water. This often needs to be repeated weekly all summer long. The baking soda will also kill some aphids. Adding soap to the spray will cause it to stick to the leaves better, making the solution much more effective. If you like you can just add some baking soda to the insecticide mix of soap and oil and have an all-around insecticide-fungicide spray mix. Unlike soap, I find that too much baking soda will damage new leaves, so stick to a maximum of six tablespoons of baking soda per gallon of water.

Do not expect these homemade sprays to be just as effective as the most powerful chemical killers. Often they're not. But they do work and they are much safer and a whole lot less likely to cause allergies.

Integrated Pest Management

Integrated Pest Management (IPM) is all about controlling pests, not about eliminating them. Using beneficial insects such as ladybugs, mealybug destroyers, tiny parasitic wasps, and green lacewings is always worth a try. It would be worthwhile for any gardener interested in allergy control to read a book or two on organic pest control. One of the better books on the subject is *The Encyclopedia of Natural Insect and Disease Control,* edited by Roger B. Yepsen, Jr. (Rodale Press, 1984). The quickest way to find sources of IPM products is to do a computer search. There are now dozens of mail order businesses that specialize in IPM.

Ants, Aphids, and Scale

Ants will farm out aphids and scale and will protect them from their natural predators. Scale are small sucking insect pests that form protective scales and live underneath them. This outer scale itself makes it difficult to control scale with conventional sprays. When the aphids and scale have ruined one part of a plant, the ants will move them to a fresh spot.

Frequently we can't seem to get rid of the insects because there are so many ants on the plants or trees. The ants will actually fight off any predatory insects that would kill the aphids or scale. I have seen ants on aphid-infested plants, warding off attacks on the aphids by ladybugs and green lacewings. With no predators, the pest insect populations quickly explode.

To kill ants I usually use a slow-acting but effective mix of powdered sugar and boric acid. Mix the sugar and boric acid fifty-fifty. Sometimes I like to flood the area where the ants are thick with a hose, and then when they're all over the place, I sprinkle the sugar and boric acid mix. You need to use caution with this method though, because boric acid contains boron, and too much of this element can be toxic to the plants themselves. Do not place this mix directly next to the trunk of small trees or vines.

A few types of ants don't much care for sugar, and for these try mixing corn meal and boric acid. This bait mix will also kill some other garden pests such as slugs, earwigs, and roaches. I have also had good luck killing ants with a mix of non-dairy creamer and boric acid. Cockroaches, by the way, inside the house can cause plenty of allergies from their dander, and the best way to kill them is with a mix of boric acid and powdered sugar as bait. Since this mix has sugar in it, it might be attractive to small children and crawling babies. Care must be taken to place it where it will be effective, but where the little kids can't get into it. Sprinkle this powder where the roaches will walk through it. You can buy boric acid in almost any drugstore. These baits are cheap, fairly safe, and they work.

The caution above concerning children also applies to pets. Don't put these baits where pets will eat them. Sometimes it works well to hide the bait under old boards or flat rocks.

Snails and Slugs

What, you may ask, do snails have to do with allergies? Well, snails or slugs will chew up plants so badly that they become weakened. Then the plants are attacked by other insects, which may lead to the growth of mold and mold spores. Where snails and slugs are common, they are a real problem. No gardener likes to see the way his or her plants look after the snails or slugs have eaten big holes in all the leaves. In California snails are almost everywhere. If you set out new transplants the snails can easily wipe them out in one or two nights. I like to grow Angel Trumpets and *Hydrangeas,* and the snails can't resist these.

So how do you control snails and slugs? I've tried, several times, putting old beer in a shallow container. Supposedly the snails love this beer and fall in and drown. Humph! Not in my yard they don't. I think they just take a drink and then go to work on my petunias. I've found a few things that do work, but not always perfectly either.

I used to go out at night with a flashlight, pick off the snails, and step on them. I know, this is messy and time-consuming, but it kills a lot of snails. I also found that snails won't cross a line of fresh wood ashes. Snails' bodies are soft and slimy, and the tiny, powdery wood ash particles stick to them and irritate them. Wood ash is also strongly alkaline, and this too negatively affects snails. Luckily I have a woodstove, and I use the ashes to protect certain plants from the snails. Once the ashes have been rained on, though, they don't work well anymore.

The old poison snail baits, which contain the chemical metaldehyde, work only so-so. Dogs often eat this stuff and die from it too, so keep that in mind. Luckily there are new and safer snail and slug bait products on the market, sold by several companies such as Garden Safe and Sluggo. The active ingredient used in these new baits is iron phosphate. Not only are the iron phosphate baits safe to use around pets, but they are also remarkably effective. If you haven't tried them yet, you'll be pleased with the results.

A Note about Ferns

Ferns don't produce mold spores, but they can produce fern spores. Often these fern spores can be just as allergenic as mold spores. Fern spores usually shoot out and land fairly close to the fern. Small ferns growing in a shady part of the garden rarely trigger allergies.

People love to grow ferns in hanging baskets, and then they often hang these over patio chairs or tables, right where someone will be sitting. Hanging basket ferns are fine, but consider the spore potential and watch where you hang them!

Tree ferns are big, robust handsome creatures, but again we need to watch where we plant them. All too often they are planted right next to front doors where they can shower spores on the people coming and going. Another consideration with tree ferns is that they have millions of tiny reddish-brown colored, needle-sharp hairs on their trunks. These little fern hairs can make you itch; they can also cause irritation of the throat and nose when they're inhaled.

The moral: Plant tree ferns back away from most human traffic. Here are some tips to keep your plants thriving:

- Keep your plants well fertilized. Without fertilizer few landscape plants will thrive. As they grow weaker, the insects start to prey on them.

- Don't overfertilize. Too much fertilizer weakens plants.

- Deep soak your trees occasionally during dry summer months. Lack of water will weaken a tree and make it a target for whiteflies, aphids, scale, spider mites, and mealybugs.

- Pay attention to pH needs of your plants. If a tree grows best on acid soil, don't plant it if your own soil is alkaline. The reverse is also true. It is difficult to get plants to thrive when the soil pH is not to their liking. If you do have acid-loving trees or shrubs growing under alkaline conditions, it will be necessary to give them additional iron in the more expensive but much more effective chelated (sequestered) form. Also, if you have acid plants in alkaline soil, they will only thrive if you lower the pH in their root zone. You can do this by using aluminum sulfate or soil sulfur at recommended rates at least once a year. If your soil is too acid for the best growth of certain of your trees or shrubs, you'll need to add lime to your soil yearly.

- Plant only smog-tolerant trees if you live in a smoggy area. If a tree is not tolerant of urban smog and it is planted right smack in the middle of a great metropolis, it will draw the pests.

- Wash down your shrubs! Get in the habit of hosing down your shrubs now and then. If you live in a smoggy or dusty area, squirt them off weekly. Dirty leaves can't take advantage of sunlight and you may end up with buggy plants.

- Keep sun-loving plants in the sun. If a hedge is made of shrubs that love bright sunshine, but someone has planted a fast-growing tree such as a pine next to them, the tree will eventually cover the shrubs in deep shade; if they live, they will certainly become an insect magnet. I know of a hedge just like this near my home. A large old hedge of lantana, now shaded by a big pine, it is literally covered top to bottom in whiteflies and mold. It is growing right outside the back entrance to a health clinic!

CHAPTER 9

Skin Rash Plants

Skin rashes caused by plants are the focus of this chapter. Many kinds of plants can cause skin rash, swelling, itching, inflammation or redness of the eyes, and other types of contact dermatitis. Often people who have no other types of allergies will nonetheless get contact dermatitis. The range of severity differs widely from one species of plant to another. Contact with some plants will cause a very short-lived, minor itchy rash, while others produce terrible, long-lasting, disfiguring rashes that turn into scars. Note that eye conditions can easily be involved if you touch the wrong plant and then rub your eyes. The wrong sort of plant sap in the eyes can and has resulted in permanent blindness.

Plant-induced dermatitis (rash) most commonly occurs on the hands, the arms, and the face, or on the legs if the gardener was wearing shorts while working in the yard. Occasionally the irritant part of the plant will actually pass through light clothing and still cause skin irritation. Patches of dermatitis may often be streaky in shape. In plant-induced dermatitis, the affected skin almost always itches; it is often red and swollen and may have blisters.

Two of the more common medical terms you will see associated with plant-caused contact rashes are "conjunctivitis" and "urticaria." Conjunctivitis is essentially swelling and/or redness of the eyelids. Urticaria is red, irritated skin rash, something similar to what you would see from contact with any of the *Urtica* species, especially the Stinging Nettles. The skin condition was essentially named after this species.

Some people are much more susceptible than others to plant-caused contact rashes. Fair-haired, light-skinned people with existing allergies to inhalant pollens are at most risk from contact allergy, but sometimes certain plants will affect almost everyone.

Not every plant-caused rash is a true allergic response. Some plants, such as common nettles, have thousands of tiny stinging hairs on their leaves and stems that can easily cause a rash, true allergy or not. But it hardly matters if the rash is an allergic response or not. It is still a rash, it is irritating, and it came from contact with the leaves, stems, flowers, roots, or sap of some plant.

People such as florists, bulb packers, and flower growers who work in the flower trades often develop allergic reactions to a good number of their own products. They often develop mysterious and diverse rashes and symptoms of the eyes, nose, throat, and respiratory system, and they may eventually have to change professions. The most common plant-caused skin rashes are from the sunflower or daisy family relatives (mums, asters, and daisies) and from the Lily family relatives (daffodils, tulips, lilies, and *Alstroemeria*).

Working with Problematic Plants

The important thing is to know which plants can cause skin problems and to then take special care when working with or around these plants. Once a person develops an allergy to contact with a particular plant, each subsequent contact will often bring a worsening of the symptoms. The only real "cure" here is to figure out which plant triggered the reaction and then to avoid any further contact with it.

There are a few precautionary things worth noting here:

- Always avoid direct skin contact with milky white "latex"-type saps such as that of the poinsettia, Natal Plum, all Spurges, and fig trees. All latex sap is highly suspect.

- When shearing or pruning, keep plant sap of any color and from any species out of your eyes. Some sap, especially that from poisonous plants, can blind you.

- Sweaty skin appears to be more susceptible to contact plant rash than dry skin.

- Since many rashes are examples of contact allergic photo-dermatitis, they will only happen, or will be worse, when the contact is made on a bright, sunny day. Some allergenic plants produce sap that sensitizes the skin to ultraviolet radiation. This can result in severe burns to a painful blistering rash in the affected areas. These blisters can develop into purplish or blackened scars. Also, bright light itself is known to worsen the skin symptoms of some individuals sensitized to plant allergens.

- Many of these allergic reactions will be "delayed." (Allergists call these delayed reactions Type IV.) Many hours or even days may pass between the time of initial contact and the breaking out of the rash or swelling. This makes it trickier to discover exactly which plant it was that affected you.

- Pollen from some large trees, oak and acacia in particular, can cause skin rash.

- Pollen from the male plants of certain separate-sexed species can cause skin rash. This is especially true with any and all male plants from the *Rhus* (poison ivy–related) family (sumac, pistache, Varnish Tree, *Cotinus,* and poison oak or poison ivy) or from the *Euphorbia* (Spurge) group. This means that you can come in contact with the plant without ever even actually touching it. You do not want any plants like this in your yard!

- Wear gloves and long-sleeved shirts when you're shearing, pruning, or otherwise working with plants that have high potential for causing rash. If you have especially sensitive skin, it would always be a good idea to wear long-sleeved shirts and sturdy gloves while you're gardening.

- Like all other types of allergy, contact allergy is often developed through overexposure over time to the same allergic plants. Thus, even though you may have worked with a certain type of plant thousands of times and never had an ill effect from it, you may eventually react to it. Actually the more you have handled a particular type of plant (if it is a potentially allergenic plant), the more susceptible you are to allergy from it.

- Many contact rash–type plants are *Euphorbia* (Spurge) relatives. This is a huge group of plants with many different species. It is important to note that all of them have latex-type sap and that the true Rubber Tree, *Hevea brasiliensis,* is also a latex-forming *Euphorbia* family member. (The houseplant rubber tree is a *Ficus,* but does have latex sap.) Anyone with the dangerous allergy to latex or rubber ought to avoid any contact with these plants. Since rubber allergy is becoming ever more common in hospitals, the use of rubber trees as hospital plants should be discouraged.

- Even though there are many allergenic plants, there are a great many more that are not, ones that do not cause allergic contact dermatitis. Not all allergenic plants cause contact dermatitis, but if you have sensitive skin, it would be a good idea to fill your gardens with plants that are allergy free.

- Not all, but a considerable number of the plants that cause severe dermatitis are also poisonous if eaten. Anyone with small children should teach them not to put plants in their mouth. Parents should keep a good list of poisonous plants handy. In chapter 10 you'll find an extensive list of poisonous plants.

- Occupational allergies are on the rise, and individuals who have hay fever or other seasonal rhinitis or asthma might want to avoid occupations such as florist, horticulturist, plant caretaker, gardener, garden worker, and plant wholesaler, all of which involve much handling of plants. People in these professions experience by far the most contact plant dermatitis.

- Those who have had numerous skin rash problems as children or teenagers, especially if their hands were involved, should probably not seek work where plants need to be handled constantly. They would just be asking for skin problems.

- To minimize their exposure to allergens, everyone working with plants should pay careful attention to washing and caring for their hands. Gloves, but not rubber gloves, should be worn whenever possible. Other work clothes should protect the skin from being scraped or scratched and from coming into contact with plant saps. Sometimes cut flowers are put in a bucket of cold water, and the water itself can easily get splashed on skin. This water has plant sap in it and may well be allergenic. Handling of plants to which you are highly sensitive should be avoided as much as possible.

- It is always a good idea for anyone who has been gardening to take a shower afterward. Allergens can often be washed off, and pollen, which easily clings to our hair, can quickly be shampooed away.

- I recommend that no one ever make cuttings of any of the *Euphorbia* family members inside a closed greenhouse unless there is an exceptional ventilation system that is running. Not only does the sap from many of these cause blistering, painful rashes, but the fumes from many are frequently allergenic and sometimes even highly carcinogenic.

Why Do Certain Plants Irritate Our Skin?

Many of the plants in the large list that follows this section will have sap that contains microscopic-sized needlelike crystals of calcium oxalate. These tiny, extremely sharp crystals can cause instantaneous and intense burning and irritation, with swelling of the lips, mouth, tongue, and pharynx if they come in contact with the mouth. This same sap can often cause skin rash as well. Oxalic acid crystals are often found in lilylike bulbs, stems, and sometimes in the leaves. This is common in many members of the large Lily and *Amaryllis* families, and also in the Arum family.

Plants with prickly leaves, like some of the juniper (especially *Juniperus communis*) and cypress trees and shrubs, can also trigger a rash. Avoid direct skin contact with prickly, itchy plants.

The fresh, clear, watery sap from the succulent stems of Jewelweed, also called Wild Impatiens, Wild Balsam, Touch-Me-Not, *Impatiens capensis,* is often useful for treating plant-caused rash. It appears to be helpful with poison ivy and poison oak rash as well. With irritation from stinging plants such as nettles, Jewelweed often provides almost instantaneous relief. Exactly how or why it works is not well understood. It was long a Native American remedy for contact with nettles and frequently grows in the same moist, wooded areas as nettles. Jewelweed grows erect, has small, trumpet-shaped orange flowers with small brown spots, and is native and common in moist areas from Alaska to Oklahoma. The ripe green seedpods burst open at the slightest touch (hence, the name Touch-Me-Nots).

Some people find relief from the itch of skin rash by applying apple cider vinegar directly to the affected area. In some cases of dermatitis the only relief comes from use of steroidal creams. Also, if you have a problem with persistent itchy skin, please see the section on the drug hydroxyzine at the end of this chapter.

One last note about the plants in this following list. I am not suggesting that gardeners do not use these plants. I'm simply saying that these plants are well documented as having caused a considerable number of contact skin and eye conditions.

Readers may go through the list and may scoff at some of the entries. "*Coleus*," someone might say, "I've worked with *Coleus* hundreds of times and never had any problem." And for them, this is no doubt perfectly true. But, nonetheless, *Coleus* is known to occasionally cause dermatitis, and that is worth knowing. Each of us is different, and we will react differently to contact with particular plants.

Years ago, when I was first teaching horticulture in a California Youth Authority (CYA) prison, I was still pretty ignorant and simplistic in my knowledge about allergies. One day I asked a student, a big, muscle-bound gangster, to weed around a clump of large perennials called Pride of Madeira *(Echium fastuosum)*. He complained that he'd done that before and that it had given him a rash.

I had worked around and handled these plants many times with no problems. I accused him of being a big wimp, and then I picked one of the large, fuzzy gray leaves and rubbed it on the inside of my forearm just to show him.

Five minutes later I had an inflamed, red, and very itchy rash on my arm. It was an eye-opener for me.

Why did this plant, which had never bothered me before, get to me this time? There could be numerous explanations: repeated exposure resulting in sensitivity, the fact that it was a hot, sunny day and I may well have been sweaty from work, or maybe it was just nature's way of showing me not to be such an ignoramus.

There are certain plants in the list below that are described as being seriously allergenic, as causing very serious rash, as having highly caustic sap. Handle these plants with extra care and consider not using them in gardens where children or pets play. The rest of them by all means do plant and enjoy. Just be aware of the unpleasant potential that they have.

Plants That Cause Skin Rash

In the following list of plants know to cause contact rashes, some of them are weeds, some are natives occasionally used in landscapes, and most are fairly common garden plants.

African Evergreen. See *Nephthytis.*

African Hemp, *Sparmannia africana,* is a houseplant that can trigger skin rash from simple contact. Rash from the sap is even more caustic.

African Milk Bush, *Synadenium grantii,* a common garden succulent type of shrubby *Euphorbia* relative, has milky latex sap that can cause very severe, dangerous skin reactions.

Agapanthus or Lily of the Nile, *Agapanthus africanus,* is a very common landscape plant in mild winter areas. Its sap, especially if in contact with a fresh scratch or an open wound, can cause long-lasting, ugly, painful skin rashes. The reaction may be either immediate or delayed.

Agave americana, **Century Plant,** a big *Agave,* is called the Century Plant because it supposedly only blooms once every one hundred years. Actually it usually blooms after only thirty years or so, and since it is monocarpic, once it blooms, it dies. Landscapers hate removing this *Agave,* in part because the huge stiff leaves are tipped with needle-sharp points.

A fiber (sisal) is made from the leaves of certain types of *Agave* and is used in making bed mattresses and sacks for shipments of coffee beans. The raw sap of the plant is corrosive to metal and highly irritating to the eyes and skin. It causes an instant, stinging red rash in gardeners who have occasion to cut any part of the plant; it also affects factory workers exposed to the sap and the wet fiber in the process of extraction. The odor of sisal in mattresses, generally in combination with some other material, causes allergic reactions in sensitive individuals. All species of *Agave* are suspect. Animals that eat *Agave* can become blind.

The sharp tips of *Agave* are perfectly capable of blinding someone should they be unlucky enough to stumble or fall into this plant. When the leaf tip pierces the skin deeply and goes in close to or against the bone, it may excite a reaction that simulates the growth of tumors. Think twice before you plant any of these in your garden.

Algerian Ivy, *Hedera canariensis*, common in mild-winter areas, has sap that causes extremely severe skin rash. This rash is almost always delayed in reaction and may not appear until days after the initial contact with the sap. Landscapers who shear back large areas of Algerian Ivy used as ground cover are especially susceptible.

***Aloe vera* and all other *Aloe* species** may seem odd to list here as plants that could cause skin rash, since *Aloe* is so popular for treating skin conditions. Perhaps it is because of this popularity that many people have long been exposed to *Aloe* sap and quite a few allergic responses are occurring. Rash from *Aloe* use is now very well documented. I have seen it myself. People prone to skin conditions in the first place might want to think twice before using *Aloe* products very often.

***Alstroemeria*, also called Peruvian Lily,** can cause lily rash. The rash from these plants began to be common in the 1990s as *Alstroemeria* have become quite popular as both garden and cut flowers. This rash is by far most common among florists or others who handle the plants often. Avoid any contact with this sap. All lily rash can be severe, and it is often very difficult to clear up.

Amaryllis **hybrids and all** *Amaryllidaceae* **members** have sap that can cause severe, long-lasting skin rash.

Anemone patens can cause contact skin rash.

Aralia **(all species)** can cause dermatitis from contact with their sap. A few species of *Aralia* can cause rash from simple contact with their flowers or leaves.

Arnica **(all species)** can cause skin rashes. They are daisy relatives.

Arrowhead Vine. See *Nephthytis.*

Arum is a large *genera* (group) of perennial plants that all have sap that can cause skin rash.

Aster **species** can all cause skin rashes from contact with their sap, leaves, or flowers. The actual symptoms may be delayed as much as several days from time of original contact with the plants. Most common in florists.

Australian Tree Ferns, *Alsophila cooperi,* can grow to almost twenty feet tall. While they're beautiful, the dead branches are covered with brown fuzz that is sharp and very itchy. The fuzz can go right through a T-shirt. Prune them with caution.

Baby's Breath, *Gypsophila paniculata,* is a very common garden plant that is used as a dried flower. When these flowers are dry, their pollen is easily released and can trigger asthma attacks. Contact with the dried flowers also can cause skin rash. Allergy to Baby's Breath is by far most common among florists and others who handle it often.

Bahia Grass and other *Paspalum* **species, which include Dallis Grass and Vasey Grass,** often have sticky seeds that can cause dermatitis.

Barbados Cherry, *Malpighia glabra,* is a tropical and Florida shrub that may have tiny stinging hairs on its leaves.

Bear Grass, *Nolina* species, are *Agave* relatives, and reactions to their sap are dangerous and very similar to that of agave. See *Agave*.

Boxwood, *Buxus japonica*, and all boxwood species have sap that can cause rash. This is most frequently seen on the hands and arms of gardeners who frequently shear boxwood hedges.

***Bryonia dioica*, also called Red Bryonia,** is a climbing herb sometimes used as an ornamental vine in mild-winter areas. Contact with the leaves, sap, and flowers causes rash.

Calla Lily, *Zantedeschia aethiopica*, is very common, and while it is a very low pollen threat plant, its sap can cause lily rash, which is often severe and hard to cure.

Candlenut. See Kukui.

Carnations, *Dianthus* species, have been known to cause rash, but this is quite rare and almost always happens only with people who handle large amounts of them daily.

Cashew tree, *Anacardium occidentale*, is a large tropical tree that produces cashew nuts. The husk that covers the nuts is highly allergenic and causes delayed poison ivy–type rash and swelling.

***Cedrela* species, Cigar Box tree and South American Cedar,** have sap that may cause blistering of skin and inflammation of eyelids. This is most common in woodworkers using this wood.

Century Plant. See *Agave americana*.

Chenille Plant, *Acalypha hispida*, is a handsome hanging houseplant that has long, feathery, red-flower clusters. Most plants in the trade are female, so there is no threat from pollen. However, these too are *Euphorbia* relatives, and their white latex sap can cause skin rash.

Chrysanthemum **species** are often implicated in contact dermatitis. All parts – flowers, stems, leaves, pollen, sap – can cause skin conditions. Reactions to *Chrysanthemum* are usually delayed and not often recognized correctly. Furthermore, light is known to worsen the skin symptoms of some individuals sensitized to *Chrysanthemum* or their relatives. This is often misdiagnosed as being caused by lupus or any number of other things.

Citrus contact (with leaves) during periods of bright sunlight can sometimes trigger episodes of photodermatitis.

Coleus **plants** *(Coleus hybridus)* have beautifully colored leaves, but contact with them does cause rash for a few gardeners. This is almost always a delayed reaction allergic response and may take several days before symptoms appear.

Cow Itch Tree. See Primrose Tree.

Crinum Lily, *Crinum zeylanicum,* sap can be very caustic and has even been known to cause skin burns on cattle.

Crotons are popular highly colored, large-leafed houseplants, but they too are *Euphorbia* relatives. Their latex sap can cause severe rash, and occasionally people will get skin rash conditions from just being around crotons.

Crown-of-Thorns, *Euphorbia milii,* is a common, thorny, red-flowered, cactuslike succulent that poses numerous allergy problems, including severe skin rash from its caustic sap.

Daffodil bulbs can cause a type of lily rash when they are handled. This is usually only seen with gardeners and people working in daffodil or narcissus packing sheds.

Dahlia **hybrids and all** *Dahlia* **species** can cause rash from contact with leaves or flowers.

***Daphne odorata* and all other *Daphne* species** are highly fragrant and especially poisonous. The plants have sap that causes severe skin rash. Rash is also possible from simple contact with the leaves.

Devil's Backbone. See Japanese Poinsettia.

Devil's Ivy, *Pothos aureus* or *Epipremnum aureum,* a common houseplant with sap that can cause rash. Watch this when making cuttings.

Devil's Maple, *Acer diabolicum,* is also called Horned Maple. The seeds have tiny, itchy, irritating hairs on them that can cause skin rash and itching.

Devil's Walking Stick, *Aralia spinosa,* like most types of *Aralia* can cause rash from contact with the leaves or flowers.

Dianthus generally causes very little allergy. However, some people have developed rashes from handling clove pinks. (Pinks are a type of *Dianthus*.)

Donkey Tail, *Euphorbia myrsinites,* causes skin rash from its latex sap. Be careful when making cuttings.

Dracaena fragrans is the most caustic of the *Dracaena* species, but all have sap that can cause severe skin rashes.

Elecampane, *Inula helenium.* See *Chrysanthemum*.

Eucalyptus – all species can cause rash and other skin eruptions from contact with their leaves and especially from their sap. Silver dollar eucalyptus leaves also cause inhalant allergies when used in dry flower arrangements.

***Euphorbia* species,** and there are thousands of them, all have latex sap, and many of them can cause serious contact dermatitis.

Feverfew. See *Chrysanthemum*. Also see Santa Maria Feverfew, *Parthenium hysterophorus*.

Fig, Fiddle Leaf Fig, *Ficus benjamina, Ficus elastica,* **and all** *Ficus* **species** have the potential for creating some problems. Contact with the rough leaves of common edible fig can cause irritation, but contact with the white latex sap from any species of *Ficus* may cause photodermatitis. This is usually a delayed reaction. This allergy is becoming considerably more common.

Freesia, an Iris family member, occasionally is implicated in causing rash on the hands of those handling the cut flowers. More common is inhalant allergy from the fragrance of freesia.

Gaillardia **species** can produce a delayed reaction–type skin rash from contact with their leaves or flowers. This is very similar to rash from chrysanthemums.

Gas Plant, *Dictamnus albus,* **and other species of** *Dictamnus* are hardy perennials from southwestern Europe, south and central Asia, Korea, and China. These plants are commonly called "burning bushes" because in dry weather flammable oil exudes from the leaves and seedpods. If a flame is placed near them, it will sometimes ignite without damaging the plant. Other common names include Dittany and Fraxinella. *D. albus* is an erect plant growing up to three feet high. The highly aromatic leaves have a sap that causes extremely severe rashes and other skin conditions. This one can cause permanent scarring and should not be used anywhere near children. The fumes from this plant are not healthy to breathe.

Geranium, *Pelargonium* **species** (all types), can cause allergic skin conditions, although this is not particularly common nor usually severe.

Gerbera Daisy or Transvaal Daisy can trigger delayed reaction–type allergic skin conditions, very similar to chrysanthemum rash.

German Ivy, *Senecio* **species** (there are many species of *Senecio*), can cause both inhalant and contact skin rash.

German Statice, *Limonium tataricum,* is often used in dried flower arrangements and can cause both inhalant and skin type allergies.

Giant Elephant Ear, *Alocasia macrorrhiza,* has a sap that is a powerful irritant.

Giant Hogweed, *Heracleum mantegazzianum,* a robust, easy-to-grow Washington State native. It is now naturalized widely, including in much of Europe. The plant exudes a clear, watery sap that sensitizes the skin to ultraviolet radiation. This can trigger severe burns to the affected areas, resulting in serious blistering and painful dermatitis. These blisters can develop into purplish or blackened scars. Giant hogweed is becoming more common in urban areas and represents an increasing public health hazard.

Ginkgo biloba fruit is not only stinky when ripe, but the juice in the fruit can cause severe skin rash. Inside the fruit are edible seeds, known as ginkgo nuts, and people who get the rash are almost always cleaning these nuts. Wear vinyl gloves for this job.

Goldenrod, *Solidago perennis,* contact can cause delayed reaction type dermatitis to people who have existing ragweed-type allergies.

Grape vines, *Vitis* **species.** Grape leaves, especially when touched on hot, sunny days, frequently cause rash for a small percentage of people. This is not normally a long-lasting rash. This rash is most common among grape pickers.

Hevea brasiliensis, **Rubber Tree,** has a sap that is especially dangerous for anyone with latex, rubber allergies. Pollen from male trees is also dangerous for people with latex allergy.

Hops Vine, *Humulus lupulus,* can cause a contact skin rash, although it is usually neither severe nor long lasting.

Horsetail, *Conyza canadensis,* has leaves and sap that may irritate skin.

Hound's Tongue or Gypsy Flower, *Cynoglossum officinale,* may cause contact dermatitis.

Japanese Poinsettia, *Pedilanthus tithymaloides,* is a houseplant with extremely caustic sap. This plant, used outside in mild winter areas, also goes under the names of redbird flower, redbird cactus, or slipper flower.

Ivy, *Hedera helix* or *Hedera canariensis.* Contact with ivy sap is well known to cause severe, painful skin rash. This is almost always a delayed-reaction response.

Kukui or Candlenut, *Aleurites moluccana,* are tall, mild-winter area trees. The raw seeds contain a powerful laxative, which is dangerous to children. Contact with candlenut latex sap can cause acute dermatitis.

Lady's Slipper, *Cypripedium calceolus,* may cause contact dermatitis.

Lagunaria patersonii. See Primrose Tree.

Leadwort, *Plumbago auriculata,* has flowers and leaves that can be a powerful irritant or may sometimes cause serious allergic reactions of the skin and eyes. All *Plumbago* species are potentially contact allergenic.

Lignum vitae or Wood of Life, *Guaiacum* **species,** is a tree or shrub whose wood is prized for its exceptional density. Exposure to toxic elements in the resin and sawdust of this wood is known to trigger sneezing and spreading contact dermatitis in woodworkers.

Malanga, *Xanthosoma* **species,** are Florida plants with irritating sap.

Mango, *Mangifera indica,* can cause rash and extreme facial swelling from contact with the leaves or the fruit and also from eating mango. People who are already sensitized to poison ivy and poison oak, mango relatives, are most likely to develop allergies to mango.

Marguerite Daisy. See *Chrysanthemum.*

Melaleuca quinquenervia **and other species of** *Melaleuca* all have oils that can be either allergenic or simply a skin irritant.

Mexican Flame Vine, *Senecio confusus,* has a sap that can cause either immediate or delayed-onset dermatitis.

Mexican Orange, *Choisya ternata,* can possibly cause photodermatitis from contact with its leaves or sap.

Mother-in-Law's Tongue, *Sansevieria trifasciata,* is an *Agave* relative and shares similar properties with its sap. See also *Agave americana.*

Motherwort, *Leonurus cardiaca,* may cause contact dermatitis.

Narcissus. See Daffodil.

Nephthytis **species, also sold as** *Syngonium podophyllum,* is an evergreen houseplant with arrow-shaped leaves. Its sap is an irritant (externally or internally) and a potential cause of dermatitis.

Nettles, Stinging Nettle, *Urtica* **species,** is common in shady, moist areas. Nettle leaves and stems are covered with tiny stinging hairs that if touched create an immediate, but short-lived, burning rash. See also Stinging Nettles.

New Zealand Flax, *Phormium tenax,* is a large, landscape perennial, popular in mild winter areas. New Zealand flax presents almost no pollen-allergy potential, but the sap from the leaves and roots is caustic and can cause serious rash. *Phormium* is an *Agave* relative. See also *Agave americana.*

Nolina texana, **Bunch Grass.** See Bear Grass.

Oak trees, *Quercus* **species,** produce large amounts of pollen that may cause dermatitis in people allergic to this pollen.

Oyster Plant, *Rhoeo spathacea,* has sap that is often highly irritating to skin.

Parthenium hysterophorus. See Santa Maria Feverfew.

Pawpaw, *Asimina triloba,* causes skin rash from the handling of unwashed pawpaw fruit.

Peace Lily, *Spathiphyllum* **species, also known as Spathe Flower, White Anthurium, or Snowflower,** is a common houseplant, and its sap is known to cause skin rash. This sap is also very irritating to the eyes.

Pepper trees, *Schinus* **species, especially the Brazilian Pepper Tree,** can cause long-lasting, blistering skin rash from contact with their leaves or especially their sap. The rash is usually delayed and is similar to rash from their relatives, poison ivy and poison oak.

Philodendron **species** have sap that can cause either immediate or delayed dermatitis.

Pickaback Plant, *Tolmiea menziesii,* **also called Piggyback Plant,** is a common houseplant that often causes contact dermatitis.

Pineapple, *Ananas comosus,* has sap in its leaves that sometimes causes rash. Some people also get skin rash from eating too much raw pineapple.

Pines, *Pinus* **species,** have tree sap that occasionally causes allergic rash. This is most common with loggers, woodworkers, and carpenters.

Plumbago. See Leadwort.

Plumeria rubra, fragrant, colorful Hawaiian plants, have a milky latex sap that can cause rash and severe irritation to the eyes. People picking the flowers from these tall plants should be careful not to let this latex drip into their eyes.

Poison ivy, poison oak, Lemonade Berry, Poison Sumac, Poison Varnish Tree, Poison Lacquer Tree, Poison Elder, Polecat Bush, Skunk Bush, Wax Tree (all are *Rhus* species) are all of extremely high contact-allergy potential. Toxins from this group may cross-react with plants in the *Schinus* genera, the pepper trees, and also with related foods such as cashews, pistachios, and especially with mangoes. Also often listed as *Toxicodendron* species.

Poisonwood, *Metopium toxiferum*, is a wild Florida plant that causes severe rash. Usually seen as a small tree or shrub, poisonwood is a relative of poison ivy, and as with all members of this Cashew family, the allergic reaction is usually delayed, sometimes for several days. All parts of the plant – leaves, stems, flowers – are allergenic.

Pride of Madeira, *Echium fastuosum*, is a large, popular, blue- or purple-flowered perennial with fuzzy gray leaves, common in mild-winter areas. Direct contact with the leaves can cause an immediate irritant rash.

Primroses, *Primula* species, are a major cause of allergic contact dermatitis. There are over four hundred species of primrose, but not all of them will cause this allergic reaction. Most allergenic are *Primula malacoides* and *Primula obconica*.

Primrose Tree, Paterson Plum, *Lagunaria patersonii*, also sometimes called Cow Itch Tree, is a mild-winter area, large evergreen tree that has beautiful pink, primrose-like flowers. The numerous seedpods of *Lagunaria* are loaded with minute, extremely sharp, stinging hairs. These can cause either immediate dermatitis if touched or inhalant allergies if inhaled.

Purple Leaf, Velvet Plant, Purple Queen, *Setcreasea purpurea*, is a common hanging houseplant with fuzzy purple leaves. Its sap is an irritant and will cause rash.

Purple Plant, *Tradescantia pallida,* is a common trailing house-plant or outdoor plant in mild winter areas. Contact can cause rash in humans and swelling and irritation in dogs and cats.

Queen Anne's Lace, *Daucus carota,* when touched during periods of bright sunlight, can cause contact photodermatitis.

Queensland Lacebark, *Brachychiton discolor,* is a mild-winter area, large ornamental tree that produces large pink flowers and very large, fuzzy, tan-colored seedpods. The fuzz that covers the seedpods is made up of millions of tiny stinging hairs that will pass right through light clothing. Rash is immediate and very irritating but not especially long-lasting.

Radish, *Raphanus sativus,* is often implicated for causing skin rash. The rash is usually triggered from touching the radish leaves, but sometimes it can also arise from eating the radishes.

***Rhus* species (all plants in this genus including sumac, Lemon-ade Berry, Varnish Tree, Sugarbush)** have highly allergenic sap that easily cross-reacts with poison ivy and poison oak sensitivities.

Rubber Tree. See *Hevea brasiliensis.* Also see Fig.

Rubber Vine, *Rhabdadenia biflora,* is a Florida plant that causes dermatitis from contact with its leaves.

Rue, *Ruta graveolens,* is a common garden herb, and contact with rue flowers, sap, or leaves often causes severe rash.

Santa Maria Feverfew, *Parthenium hysterophorus,* is a common weed along the Gulf Coast and in Mexico, and now also in some other countries such as India. Contact can cause very severe rash. The pollen of this plant is also exceptionally allergenic. Rash may be immediate (Type I) or may be delayed for up to forty-eight hours (Type IV).

***Sapium* species** are often large trees, separate-sexed, and are

Euphorbia relatives. Their sap can cause rash and is of special concern to those with allergy to rubber (latex), as is the sap of any and all *Euphorbia* species.

Schefflera. See Umbrella Tree.

Shell Flower or Shell Ginger, *Alpinia* species, have leaves and sap that cause dermatitis.

Showy Lady's-Slipper, *Cypripedium reginae,* is a native orchid found in eastern Canada. Lady's-slipper can cause dermatitis in sensitive individuals with symptoms quite similar to those of poison ivy.

Silk Oak, *Grevillea robusta,* a common large, fast-growing landscape tree in mild-winter areas, has sap that is highly irritating to skin.

Snake Plant. See Mother-in-Law's Tongue.

Snowdrop, a garden perennial planted from bulbs, has properties similar to those found in daffodils. Its sap can cause rash.

Spathe Flower. See Peace Lily.

Squill, *Scilla* species, can trigger skin rash in people handling the *Scilla* bulbs.

***Sterculia* species,** trees that are used in Florida and tropical landscapes, have stinging hairs around their seeds that cause immediate irritation.

Stinging Nettles, *Urtica dioica,* give instant pain and a short-lived rash from their tiny, sharp stinging plant hairs. Rash and the pain are caused by the puncturing of the skin from the hairs and from histamine-like compounds on the stems and leaves.

Sunflower, *Helianthus annuus,* occasionally causes skin rashes. Reactions are usually delayed, rarely immediate.

Sycamore trees, *Platanus* species, all have tiny hairs on their fuzzy leaves. These hairs can cause both inhalant problems and skin rash.

Tomato plant stems and leaves occasionally trigger a short-lived skin rash. This same rash can also be found among food workers who have to slice many tomatoes.

***Toxicodendron* species, poison ivy, poison oak, Poison Sumac.** All have Type IV delayed reactions. Contact with any part of these plants – leaves, stems, roots, flowers, and pollen – can cause rash. See also *Rhus* species.

Tread-Softly, *Cnidoscolus urens,* a curiosity greenhouse plant, has stinging hairs that cause instant rash on contact.

Tree Ferns. See Australian Tree Ferns.

Tree-of-Heaven, *Ailanthus altissima,* a common, weedy tree sometimes also known as stink tree, occasionally causes rash from contact with its odd-smelling leaves.

Trumpet Creeper, *Campsis radicans,* is a common, hardy flowering vine that is also called the cow-itch vine. Contact with the leaves or flowers can cause itching and rash.

Tulip bulbs when handled frequently cause symptoms known as "tulip finger," a kind of lily rash.

Umbrella Tree, *Schefflera, Brassaia actinophylla,* occasionally causes dermatitis from contact with its sap or leaves.

Vanilla Vine, *Vanilla planifolia,* a tropical or greenhouse plant, has sap that can cause dermatitis.

Varnish Tree, *Rhus verniciflua,* is a landscape tree that can cause severe dermatitis from contact with its sap, flowers, pollen, or leaves. Reactions will almost always be delayed. This is typical for *Rhus* species, which are all poison ivy relatives.

Virgin's Bower, *Clematis virginiana*, may cause contact skin rash.

Wafer Ash, *Ptelea baldwinii*, causes photosensitization (making one more sensitive to sunlight) and contact dermatitis.

Wild parsnip, *Pastinaca sativa*, can cause rash from handling of the leaves or roots.

Windflower, *Anemone* species, can cause rash and irritation from contact with any part of the plant.

Yarrow. See *Chrysanthemum.*

Yellow Iris, *Iris pseudacorus*, is a naturalized plant found in wet areas. This poisonous plant has sap that can cause dermatitis in sensitive humans.

Yellow Lady's Slipper. See Lady's Slipper.

Zulu Potato, *Bowiea volubilis*, also called Climbing Onion, is a greenhouse plant that can cause contact rash.

An Old but Useful Drug for Relief of Itching?

I am not in the habit of recommending particular medications since I am not a physician and drugs are not my area of expertise. However, I would like to draw attention to hydroxyzine, a prescription drug that has been on the market since 1953. Hydroxyzine was originally developed as an anti-anxiety drug, but it was soon discovered that it often was very effective at stopping itching.

Perhaps because this drug has been around a long time and is no longer under patent, it does not appear to me to be recommended by doctors as often as it perhaps should be. Hydroxyzine (pronounced hi DROX i zeen), which may be sold under many different trade names, is inexpensive, and I have personally seen it work very well with persistent itchy skin rashes when no other drug did. Some names hydroxyzine has been sold under include Apo-Hydroxyzine, Atarax, Marax (CD), Marax DF (CD), Multi-pax, Vistaril, and Vistrax (CD).

Side effects from this drug also appear to be modest, although it does have a sedative effect and would impair doing some things like driving cars or flying airplanes.

As anyone who ever gets rashes knows only too well, most rashes itch something terrible, and the more you scratch them, the worse they often get. Thus getting rid of the itch is often necessary to be rid of that irritating rash.

Ask your own doctor about hydroxyzine.

CHAPTER 10

Poisonous Plants and Poisonous Pollen

I'd like to pass on a true story about my own daughter Naomi. The spring we moved into the house that we now live in, Naomi, about age nine then, was constantly sick with a terrible sore throat. We took her to several doctors and an allergist, and none of them came up with anything. She was sick for almost three months and then started to get better. By summer she was perfectly okay.

The next spring the same thing happened all over again and we took her to new doctors. Nothing helped, but by summer she was fine.

The third spring the exact same thing happened again. Naomi was sick and feeling miserable with a sore throat and constant coughing.

One day my eight-year-old son, Josh, and I were out in our backyard playing wiffleball. Josh was a strong kid and a great hitter.

He smacked one ball hard, and it went foul, straight into this large Yew Pine *(Podocarpus macrophyllus)* shrub that grew right next to Naomi's bedroom. The wiffleball hit smack in the middle of the bush, and a big cloud of "smoke" flew up from the Yew Pine.

"Look, Josh," I told him, "look at all that pollen!" Now, Josh was my son, of course, and had been growing up in a house where his father was both a horticulturist and an allergy researcher.

"Is that a male tree?" he asked me.

I sheepishly admitted that it was indeed a male.

"Then what is it doing in our yard?" he asked me.

I was staggered, and embarrassed too. I had left that shrub growing there because it was a handsome plant, and even though I knew it was male, at that point in my research I had yet to document allergy caused by Yew Pines. But nonetheless, it was a pollen-producing male, and it certainly had no place in my backyard.

"Okay, Josh," I told him, "when we're done playing ball, we'll get rid of it."

And that's what we did. We chopped it down and dug up the stump and roots. Not long after, I replaced it with a perfect-flowered guava bush.

Naomi's symptoms disappeared, but I didn't make the connection. Several years later I mentioned the wiffleball story to a friend of mine, and my wife, Yvonne, said, "You know, Tom, since you and Josh cut down that bush, Naomi has never had that terrible sore throat again."

I now know better about Yew Pine pollen. It is a yew relative, and like the yews *(Taxus* species), all parts of it are quite poisonous, including the pollen. Allergists almost never skin test for yew or *Podocarpus* pollen since they usually only have their pollen monitoring equipment way up high on buildings, typically on the third floor roof of a hospital. Yew or *Podocarpus* pollen is fairly dense and is rarely found up there. But it is perfectly common down where we live.

Naomi never did get those sore throats again. Several springs ago I was in Los Angeles doing some talks, and I stayed with friends who lived there. They asked me to look over their yard for its allergy potential. The first thing I noticed was that the large tree overhanging the entire front porch was a Fern Pine *(Podocarpus gracilior)*. It was a male tree, and it was loaded with pollen cones. When I shook the tip of a branch, a cloud of pollen arose. On both sides of their bedroom, Yew Pines had been planted as foundation shrubs. (Both the Fern Pine and Yew Pines were litter-free, fruitless male plants.) This use of Yew Pines and Fern Pines as foundation shrubs is a very common practice in warm areas, much as it is a common landscape practice in cold-winter areas to use yews *(Taxus* species) as foundation plants. Yews, like *Podocarpus,* are separate sexed, and the males have pollen that is poisonous.

I told my friends about Naomi, and it turned out that they too had both been having the same symptoms themselves – for the past five years, every spring. The solution was the axe, and this they did a week later. This last spring I talked to them, and for the first time in the past six years, they had not been sick. The sore throats were a thing of the past.

Toxic Pollen or Allergenic Pollen, or Both?

In the last few years I have become increasingly concerned about the effects of breathing in poisonous pollen. This is far more common than you might think.

There is often some confusion about the differences in the terms "allergenic" and "poisonous." An allergenic substance will only affect those who are allergic to it. Olive tree pollen is not poisonous, but it can trigger allergic responses in many people with allergies who happen to inhale it. Pollen from yew *(Taxus* species) is poisonous. If inhaled, yew pollen can make anyone sick, whether they have allergies or not. A poisonous substance is toxic, and it will have a negative health effect on anyone who eats, inhales, or injects it. Poison pollen can affect anyone, but it will have the most severe effects on young children, the elderly, anyone with a tendency to asthma or pneumonia, and on anyone whose immune system is compromised.

This chapter, on poisonous plants, is included because too few horticultural books have decent lists of these. Since the aim of *Safe Sex in the Garden* is to combine botany, horticulture, and health, a frank discussion of poisonous plants is in order. Please note: A substance that is poisonous is not necessarily allergenic. A substance that is allergenic is certainly not necessarily poisonous; however, there are certain substances that are both allergenic and poisonous. These would usually be certain types of pollen from poisonous plants.

Plants may be entirely poisonous, as with an oleander, or they may simply have certain parts that are poisonous. For example, every part of a yew is poisonous except for its ripe red fruit. Another example of this would be rhubarb, where the leaves are poisonous but the stems are edible.

There can be parallels between the side effects people experience with chemotherapy and the effects of people exposed to large amounts of poisonous pollen. (It is worth noting that Taxol, a chemotherapy drug, is made from yew trees.) In chemo the patient is given doses of poison large enough to kill off their cancer cells but hopefully not to kill the patient. The side effects of chemo are many, and almost all of them, as can be expected from poisoning, are most unpleasant. Typical negative health effects of inhaling poisonous pollen are sore throat, headache, nausea, lethargy, irritability, and coughing or tightness in the chest.

Pollen of some species is actually edible and is considered by some to be a health tonic. However, pollen from most highly poisonous plants is poisonous. Inhaling poisons can just as easily poison us as eating them could. Actually substances that are inhaled are almost always more dangerous than those same substances would be if we ate them. Our stomach acids are able to break down many types of poisons that our mucous membranes are not.

In the list of poisonous plants below, the most highly poisonous, the most deadly, will be marked with a skull and crossbones. However, all of these plants listed are indeed poisonous, and if enough plant material is eaten, death can result. The actual amount that would have to be eaten to result in death will vary widely from species to species. Again, the most at risk are the very young, the very weak, and those who are already ill. Still, these are poisonous plants, and with many of them, even a tiny amount, a leaf, a few seeds, the toxicity is powerful enough that it could kill a perfectly healthy adult if ingested.

There are a few plants in this list that are not especially toxic to humans but that are quite toxic to pets, such as dogs, cats, or horses. Most, but not all, plants that are toxic to humans would also be toxic to dogs or cats. In addition, almost any plant that is marked with skull and crossbones would more than likely also be toxic for large animals such as cattle, sheep, and horses.

Nursery Plant Tags

I would like to propose something here, a simple, logical idea suggested to me recently in an email from a young lady studying landscape design in San Diego. She asked me, "Why is it that poisonous plants for sale are not labeled that they are poisonous?"

Small children often stick odd things in their mouths, and as a result they are especially at risk from poisonous plants. This is something every one of us ought to be concerned about. If a plant is poisonous, when it is sold the plant tag should make note of this. Usually, though, this is not the case. If a plant, for example, with poisonous pollen were planted next to an asthmatic child's window, this could have extremely serious affects. Toddlers who stick highly poisonous plants in their mouths could die. Nursery plants that are poisonous need to be tagged clearly stating this important fact. I encourage all readers to talk to nurserypeople about the need for this, write to your elected representatives and ask them to mandate this, send emails and letters to the editor about this. Let's all promote this idea.

A few more comments about the list below: One of my editors who read this chapter scribbled a note saying, "Just what are readers supposed to do with this – not plant avocados, amaryllis, Angel Trumpets? Clematis?"

Another editor suggested that I "only include the most deadly plants, the ones that are listed with the skull and crossbones."

I prefer to leave the list as is for several reasons. First, we who garden and buy books about gardening are often the first people who will be asked for advice if a child has eaten some odd plant.

Second, some people have implied that my writing gives the wrong message about plants, that plants can cause allergies or illness. Well, the truth is some plants can be dangerous to our health. Ignorance is not bliss. Let's have all the facts.

Third, I have never intended that readers should not grow any plants that are poisonous or allergenic. Grow whatever you like! But by being armed with correct health information about plants, we can make the most rational choices as to where to plant something, how many to plant, which ones to be the most alert about.

Finally, I admit this list is huge, but keep in mind that in North America alone, we use more than twenty thousand different species of plants in our gardens and landscapes. In addition there are un-counted thousands of additional varieties, cultivars, subspecies, and unusual forms. Compared to the actual number of different plants involved, perhaps this list will not seem so large.

Poison Control Centers

Each state in the United States has a poison control center where you can call for fast, free advice. (When I called the California poison control center recently, the phone was answered by an M.D., too.) Look in the Emergency Crisis Hotlines section of your local white pages for your state's center's phone number. You can also call 1-800-222-1222, and your call will be routed to your local poison control center.

Poisonous Plants

Those marked with the skull and crossbones are especially lethal.

Aconite, *Aconitum* species ☠

African Evergreen, *Syngonium podophyllum*

African Milk Bush, *Synadenium grantii* ☠

Algerian Ivy, *Hedera canariensis*

Amaryllis, Naked Lady, *Amaryllis belladonna*

Anemone, Windflower, *Anemone* species ☠

Angel Trumpet, *Brugmansia* species or *Datura* species

Arnica, *Arnica montana* ☠

Arrowgrass, *Triglochin maritimum*

Atamasca Lily or Rain Lily, *Zephyranthes atamasca* ☠

Aucuba japonica, Gold Dust Plant

Autumn Crocus, *Colchicum autumnale* ☠

Avocado, *Persea americana* (leaves poisonous)

Azalea indica, and all other species ☠

Baneberry, *Actaea* species

Beard Tongue, *Penstemon* species

Belladonna, *Atropa bella-donna* ☠

Be Still Plant, Yellow Oleander, Lucky Nut, *Thevetia peruviana* ☠

Bird Cherry, Sweet Cherry, *Prunus avium* (broken seeds, twigs, leaves poisonous) ☠

Black-Eyed Susan, *Rudbeckia serotina*

Black Jetbead, *Rhodotypos scandens* ☠

Black Locust, *Robinia pseudoacacia*

Bleeding Heart, *Dicentra* species ☠

Bloodroot, *Sanguinaria canadensis*

Bouncing Bet, *Saponaria* species

Boxwood, *Buxus* species

Bracken Fern, *Pteridium aquilinum* ☠

Buckeye, *Aesculus* species ☠

Buckwheat, *Fagopyrum esculentum*

Buttercups or Crowfoot, *Ranunculus* species ☠

Butterfly Weed, *Asclepias tuberosa*

Caladium, *Caladium bicolor*

Calla Lily, *Calla* species or *Zantedeschia aethiopica*

Canada Moonseed, *Menispermum* species ☠

Carolina Cherry Laurel, *Prunus caroliniana* ☠

Carolina Jessamine, *Gelsemium sempervirens* ☠

Cassia or Senna, *Cassia* species

Castor Bean, *Ricinus communis* ☠

Celandine, *Chelidonium majus* ☠

Chalice Vine, *Solandra guttata* ☠

Cherimoya, *Annona cherimola* (seeds poisonous) ☠

Cherries, Black Cherry, Bitter Cherry, Chokecherry, and Pin Cherry, *Prunus* species (leaves, seeds poisonous) ☠

Chinaberry Tree, *Melia azedarach*

Chinese Scholar Tree, *Sophora japonica*

Chinese Tallow Tree, *Sapium sebiferum*

Chives, *Alium* species (can be poisonous to dogs and cats)

Christmas Rose, *Helleborus niger*

Clematis, Virgin's Bower, *Clematis hybrida* and other species

Cocklebur, *Xanthium strumarium*

Coltsfoot, *Tussilago farfara* (may cause cancer)

Coontie, *Zamia pumila*

Coral plant, *Jatropha multifida* (seeds poisonous, pollen also poisonous) ☠

Coral Tree, Coral Bean, *Erythrina* species (seeds poisonous)

Corn Cockle, *Agrostemma githago*

Corn Lily, False Hellebore, *Veratrum californicum* ☠

Cow Cockle, *Saponaria* species

Crape Myrtle, *Lagerstroemia indica*

Creeping Charlie, *Glechoma* species or *Pilea* species

Croton, *Codiaeum variegatum*

Crown-of-Thorns, *Euphorbia milii* ☠

Crown Vetch, *Coronilla varia*

Cycas Palms, Sago Palm, *Cycas* species

Cyclamen, *Cyclamen persicum* (root poisonous)

Daffodil, *Narcissus pseudonarcissus* ☠

Daphne, *Daphne* species ☠

Day-Blooming Jasmine, *Cestrum diurnum* (fruits poisonous)

Death Angel Mushrooms, *Amanita* species ☠

Death Camas, *Zigadenus* species ☠

Death Cap Mushrooms, *Amanita* species ☠

Delphiniums, Larkspur, *Delphinium* species ☠

Devil's Trumpet, *Datura* species

Dock, Curly Dock, *Rumex* species

Dogbane, *Apocynum* species ☠

Doll's-Eyes, *Actaea* species

Drooping Leucothoe, *Leucothoe axillaris* ☠

Dumb Cane, *Dieffenbachia bausei*

Dutchman's Breeches, Bleeding Hearts, *Dicentra* species ☠

Earthstar, *Scleroderma geaster* ☠

Elderberry, *Sambucus rubra* (leaves, bark, and roots are poisonous) ☠

Elephant's Ear, *Colocasia* species

English Ivy, *Hedera helix*

English Laurel, *Prunus laurocerasus* ☠

Ephedra species (can be toxic to small animals)

Erica, *Erica* species ☠

Euphorbia, Spurge, all species ☠

European Bittersweet, *Solanum dulcamara* ☠

European Spindle Tree, *Euonymus europaea* ☠

False Sego Palm or False Sago Palm, *Cycas* species

Fern Pine, *Podocarpus gracilior* ☠

Fescue Grass, *Festuca* species (can be poisonous to sheep, cattle, and horses)

Fetterbush, *Pieris japonica* ☠

Fetterbush, Stagger plant, Maleberry, *Lyonia* species ☠

Fiddleneck, *Amsinckia intermedia*

Figwort, *Scrophularia nodosa*

Fishtail Palm, *Caryota mitis* (fruit poisonous)

Flamingo Lily, *Anthurium andraeanum*

Flax, *Linum usitatissimum* (immature seedpods are poisonous)

Forget-Me-Not, *Myosotis scorpioides* (can cause liver cancer if eaten in quantity)

Four-o-Clock, *Mirabilis jalapa*

Foxglove, *Digitalis purpurea* ☠

Frangipani, *Plumeria* species

Garlic (poisonous to dogs and cats)

Gold Dust Plant, *Aucuba japonica*

Golden Chain or Laburnum, *Laburnum anagyroides* ☠

Golden Dew Drop, Pigeon Berry, *Duranta repens*

Goldenrod, *Solidago,* all species

Golden Shower tree, *Cassia fistula*

Gopher Plant, *Euphorbia lathyrus* ☠

Great Lobelia, Cardinal Flower, Indian Tobacco, *Lobelia* species

Ground Ivy, Creeping Charlie, Gill-over-the-Ground, *Glechoma* species

Groundsels, *Senecio* species

Halogeton, *Halogeton glomeratus*

Hellebore, *Veratrum viride*

Henbane, *Hyoscyamus niger* ☠

Holly, *Ilex* species (berries poisonous)

Horsebrush, *Tetradymia* species

Horse Chestnut, *Aesculus* species ☠

Horse Nettle, *Solanum* species

Horsetail, *Equisetum arvense* and other species

Hyacinth, *Hyacinthus* species

Hydrangea, *Hydrangea macrophylla* (leaves poisonous)

Indian Pink, *Spigelia marilandica* ☠

Iris, *Iris,* all species

Ivy, English, Baltic, or Algerian, *Hedera* species

Jack-in-the-Pulpit, *Arisaema* species

Japanese Euonymus, *Euonymus japonica*

Japanese Pieris, *Pieris japonica* and other species ☠

Jatropha species, especially *Jatropha curcas* ☠

Java Bean, Lima Bean, *Phaseolus lunatus* (raw beans poisonous) ☠

Jerusalem Cherry, *Physalis* species (unripe fruit poisonous) ☠

Jerusalem Cherry, *Solanum pseudocapsicum*

Jessamine, *Gelsemium sempervirens* ☠

Jetberry Bush, *Rhodotypos scandens* ☠

Jimsonweed, *Datura* species

Kaffir Lily, *Clivia miniata*

Kalmia, Mountain Laurel, *Kalmia* species ☠

Kentucky Coffee Tree, *Gymnocladus dioica*

Klamath Weed, *Hypericum perforatum*

Kochia, *Kochia scoparia*

Lamb's Quarters, *Chenopodium album*

Lantana, Red Sage, Yellow Sage, or West Indian, *Lantana camara* ☠

Larkspur, *Delphinium* species ☠

Laurel Snailseed, *Cocculus laurifolius* ☠

Ligustrum species, Privets (all parts poisonous, especially seeds) ☠

Lily, *Lilium* species

Lily-of-the-Valley, *Convallaria majalis* ☠

Lupine, *Lupinus* species

Maleberry, Fetterbush, *Lyonia* species ☠

Marsh Marigold or Cowslip, *Caltha palustris*

Mayapple or Mandrake, *Podophyllum peltatum* ☠

Melia, Chinaberry, *Melia* species

Mexican Poppy, *Argemone mexicana*

Mexican Tea, *Chenopodium ambrosioides* ☠

Milkweed, *Asclepias* species

Mistletoe, *Phoradendron* species

Monkey Agaric Mushrooms, *Amanita* species ☠

Monkshood, *Aconitum* species ☠

Moonseed, *Menispermum canadense* ☠

Morning Glory, *Ipomoea* species

Mountain Fetterbush, *Pieris japonica* and other species ☠

Mountain Laurel, *Kalmia* species ☠

Mountain Mahogany, *Cercocarpus* species ☠

Narcissus. See Daffodil ☠

Necklace Pod, *Sophora tomentosa* ☠

Night-Blooming Jasmine, *Cestrum nocturnum*

Nightshade, Black Nightshade, or Deadly Nightshade,
    Atropa bella-donna ☠

Oak trees, *Quercus* species

Oleander, *Nerium oleander* ☠

Onions, *Alium* species (poisonous to some small animals,
    especially to cats)

Panther Cap Mushrooms, *Amanita* species ☠

Peace Lily, *Spathiphyllum* species

Peach, plum, cherry, nectarine, *Prunus* species (seeds, twigs,
    leaves poisonous) ☠

Penciltree, *Euphorbia* species ☠

Penstemon, Beard Tongue, *Penstemon* species

Peony, *Paeonia* species

Peperomia, *Peperomia obtusifolia*

Periwinkle, *Catharanthus roseus*

Pernettya, *Pernettya* species (*Gaultheria* species) ☠

Philodendrons, all species (especially toxic for cats)

Pigweed, *Amaranthus* species

Pin Cherry, *Prunus pensylvanica* (seeds, twigs, leaves
    poisonous) ☠

Podocarpus, *Podcarpus* species ☠

Poinsettia, *Euphorbia pulcherrima*

Poinsettia, *Euphorbia* species

Poison Hemlock, *Conium maculatum* ☠

Poison Ivy, *Toxicodendron radicans*

Poison Oak, *Toxicodendron diversilobum*

Poison Sumac, *Toxicodendron vernix*

Pokeweed, Poke, Poke Salad, *Phytolacca americana* ☠

Pomegranate, *Punica granatum* (bark poisonous)

Ponderosa Pine, *Pinus ponderosa* (poisonous to cattle only)

Poppies, including Opium Poppy, *Papaver* species ☠

Potato, *Solanum* species (green parts of tubers and sprouts poisonous) ☠

Prickly Poppy, *Argemone mexicana*

Privet, *Ligustrum* species (seeds poisonous) ☠

Purple Sesbane, *Sesbania punicea* or *Daubentonia punicea* (seeds poisonous) ☠

Quailbush, *Atriplex lentiformis* and other species ☠

Queen Palm, *Arecastrum romanzoffianum* (green seeds poisonous)

Ragweed, *Ambrosia* species

Ragworts, *Senecio* species

Rain Lily, *Zephyranthes atamasca* ☠

Red Elderberry, *Sambucus canadensis*

Red Maple, *Acer rubrum* (usually affects horses only)

Red Mulberry, *Morus rubra* (unripe fruit poisonous)

Rhododendron, *Rhododendron* species

Rhubarb, *Rheum rhaponticum* (leaves poisonous)

Rock Poppy, Celandine, *Chelidonium majus* ☠

Rosary Pea, *Abrus precatorius* ☠

Rue, *Ruta graveolens* ☠

Sago Palm, *Cycas revoluta*

Saint John's Wort, *Hypericum perforatum*

Sapodilla, *Manilkara zapota* (seeds and bark poisonous)

Sapote, *Casimiroa edulis* (seeds poisonous)

Scarlet Pimpernel, *Anagallis arvensis*

Scilla, all species

Scotch Broom, *Cytisus scoparius* ☠

Senecio, *Senecio* species

Sensitive Fern, *Onoclea sensibilis*

Service Berry, Shadblow, *Amelanchier alnifolia* (poisonous to sheep, goats, and cattle only)

Siberian Squill, *Scilla* species ☠

Sierra Laurel, *Leucothoe davisiae* ☠

Silk Oak, *Grevillea robusta*

Skullcap, *Scutellaria lateriflora*

Skunk Cabbage, *Symplocarpus foetidus*

Snailseed, *Cocculus laurifolius* ☠

Sneezeweed, *Helenium autumnale* (especially poisonous for dogs)

Snowberry, *Symphoricarpos* species

Snowdrop, *Galanthus nivalis*

Snow-on-the-Mountain, *Euphorbia* species ☠

Soapberry Tree, *Sapindus saponaria*

Sorghum (can poison cows, sheep, and horses)

Spanish Bayonet, *Yucca aloifolia* (roots poisonous)

Spanish Broom, *Cytisus* species ☠

Spathe Flower, *Spathiphyllum* species

Spider Lily, *Hymenocallis* species, or *Lycoris radiata* (bulbs poisonous)

Spider Plant, *Chlorophytum comosum* (toxic for cats)

Spindle Tree, *Euonymus* species ☠

Spurges, *Euphorbia* species ☠

Squill, *Scilla* species ☠

Squirrel Corn, *Dicentra* species ☠

Star-of-Bethlehem, *Ornithogalum umbellatum*

Stinging Nettle, *Urtica* species

Sudan Grass (can poison cows, sheep, and horses)

Sugar Apple, *Annona squamosa* (seeds very poisonous) ☠

Sweet Clover, *Melilotus alba* and *Melilotus officinalis*

Sweet Coltsfoot, *Petasites hybridus* (cancerous in large doses)

Sweet Pea, Tangier Pea, Everlasting Pea, Oregon Wild
Sweet Pea, Caley Pea, and Singletary Pea, *Lathyrus*
species

Sweetshrub, *Calycanthus floridus*

Sweet Woodruff, *Asperula odorata*

Swiss Cheese Plant, *Monstera deliciosa*

Tall Fescue, *Festuca arundinacea*

Tansy, *Tanacetum vulgare*

Tartarian Honeysuckle, *Lonicera tatarica*

Thornapple, *Argemone mexicana*

Tobacco and Tree Tobacco, *Nicotiana* species ☠

Tulip, *Tulipa* species

Tung Oil Tree, *Aleurites fordii* ☠

Umbrella Tree, *Brassaia actinophylla*

Velvet Bean, *Mucuna* species ☠

Velvet Plant, Purple Velvet Plant, *Setcreasea purpurea*

Venus Flytrap, *Dionaea* species

Vetch, Hairy Vetch, Narrow-Leafed Vetch, Purple Vetch,
Broad Beans, *Vicia* species

Viburnum, *Viburnum* species (uncooked fruits are
poisonous)

Vinca major, Vinca minor

Vipers Bugloss, *Echium plantagineum*

Virginia Creeper, *Parthenocissus quinquefolia* (berries
poisonous) ☠

Wallflower, *Cheiranthus cheiri*

Walnut, *Juglans* species (walnut wood shavings can poison horses)

Water Hemlock or Cowbane, *Cicuta* species ☠

Watermelon Begonia, *Pilea cadierei*

White Sapote, *Casimiroa edulis* (seeds poisonous)

White Snakeroot, *Eupatorium rugosum* ☠

Windflower, *Anemone* species

Winter Cress, *Barbarea vulgaris*

Wintersweet, *Acokanthera* species

Wisteria Vine, *Wisteria* species

Wolfsbane, *Aconitum* species ☠

Wormseed, Mexican Tea, *Chenopodium ambrosioides* ☠

Wormwood, *Artemisia absinthium*

Yellow Allamanda, *Allamanda cathartica*

Yellow Oleander, *Thevetia peruviana* ☠

Yellow Star Thistle, *Centaurea solstitialis*

Yesterday, Today, and Tomorrow, *Brunfelsi americana*

Yew, *Taxus cuspidata* or any other *Taxus* species ☠

Yew Pine, *Podocarpus macrophyllus* and other species ☠

Zephyr Lily, Rain Lily, Fairy Lily, Atamasca Lily, *Zephyranthes atamasca* ☠

CHAPTER 11

Animal Allergies

Yes, pets have allergies – often very serious allergies. Almost any plant allergen that is a problem in human allergies is also of potential concern in animal allergies. Our pets spend much time outside, and they are constantly exposed to pollen and mold spores. They are closer to the ground, and their fur often traps a good deal of pollen.

Unfortunately a dog or cat can't tell us that he or she is experiencing hay fever or asthma, but if we know what to look for we can figure it out. Often it's the same sort of allergy symptoms we humans experience – sneezing, red or runny eyes, coughing, and itching can all be signs that a dog, cat, or other animal is experiencing allergies. But not always. Read on.

Don't Always Blame the Dog

In many cases pets, dogs especially, are blamed for the allergies of their owners, and in many cases the blame is misplaced. (Pollen from allergenic plants growing in the back yard will easily get trapped in a dog's hair.) People, who then come in contact with the dog, come in contact with this pollen. They blame the dog when it is really the plants growing in their yard.

Not long ago, after one of my talks to a group of Master Gardeners, a woman from the audience came up to buy a book. Then she told me a story I'm sure I'll never forget. During my talk I had told them about the very first sniff tests I had done on people and the incredibly powerful reactions some of them had from sniffing bottlebrush flowers. (Bottlebrush is a type of myrtle.) I explained that looking at this bottlebrush pollen under a microscope, I'd discovered that it was tiny, profuse, sticky, and shaped just like minute ninja stars. The pollen grains of this species were all triangular, and each point was so acute that it was needle sharp. Obviously bottlebrush pollen would easily stick in the mucous membranes and could aggravate the sinuses simply by mechanical action. It was, of course, also quite allergenic.

Bottlebrush is one of many plants that have pollen that, because of its shape, won't travel far in the air. To get a dose of pollen like this you usually need to be very close to the bush itself.

The woman from the audience told me, "We used to have this wonderful family dog – a big, friendly golden retriever. I loved him, and so did my husband and our kids. We really loved this dog, but when he came in the house he would shake himself, and everyone near him would start sneezing. It just got worse and worse. Eventually we decided," she told me, "that we had to get rid of him, much as we hated to do it."

I didn't even want to ask how they'd gotten rid of him.

"Our dog," she explained to me, "had a favorite spot out in the backyard where he would always sleep or just go to get out of the sun. It was right in the middle of a big bottlebrush shrub."

She had suddenly realized as I was speaking that their dog must have been getting that sticky pollen all over him from that bottlebrush. When he came inside and shook himself, everyone near him got a quick blast of bottlebrush pollen. Since these shrubs will flower for many months on end, this probably happened many times over.

"If only we'd had known," she said. "We would have gotten rid of that bush and kept our poor dog."

I would expect also that the dog himself had probably developed an allergy to the bottlebrush pollen. This is probably why he tried to shake himself clean of it. The pollen was irritating to him too.

Common Allergies for Common Pets

Almost any kind of pet can have allergies, but certain allergies are more common with one type of animal than another. Pollen from male ash trees, for example, will set dogs and cats up for later allergy from pollen of the ash relatives, such as the olives and privets. With most of our pets, be they rabbits, parrots, dogs, or cats, exposure to too much pollen or mold can and will cause allergies. Later in this chapter we'll discuss treatment of these allergies.

CATS AND DOGS

Cats, because they lick themselves so often, are especially susceptible to all kinds of insecticides, fungicides, and herbicides. It is important to remember that exposure to these chemical pesticides can harm the immune systems of our pets and make allergies much more likely to happen. Lawn products such as weed and feed (a mix of fertilizer and lawn herbicide) should be used sparingly, if at all, on lawns where our pets play and sleep. Any chemical product used to kill dandelions or other lawn weeds may be quite harmful to our cats.

Dogs are much more susceptible to allergies than are cats. Certain breeds of dogs tend to have more allergies than others. Those considered most susceptible are Skye terriers, Scottish terriers, and Boston terriers, golden retrievers, Irish setters, German shepherds, West Highland white terriers, miniature schnauzers, shar-peis, shih tzus, pugs, poodles, and dalmatians. Mutts are the least susceptible. Mutts are often generally healthier than purebreds for two reasons. First, they are not inbred, which can bring out any inheritable weaknesses. Second, they are often crosses of two purebred parents, and this results in what animal breeders call "hybrid vigor." Usually a dog will not show any signs of allergies until it is between one and three years old, no matter the breed. It usually takes five to seven years of exposure to an allergen for a person to develop a particular allergy, but with a dog everything happens quicker.

Dogs that are kept inside all the time can sometimes become allergic to dander from their human owners. Dogs can also become allergic to cat dander. While cats can also become allergic to dander from dogs, this is much more rare than the reverse.

BIRDS

While odors and fragrances may well bother people and mammals, birds are especially allergic to strong smells. Birds are also especially sensitive to fumes from smoke, and even more so to fumes from chemicals such as pesticides, fungicides, and herbicides. The coal miners didn't take a canary down in the mine with them for nothing. Parrots have died from the fumes when their owners burned a Teflon-coated frying pan. Anyone raising birds, parrots and parakeets especially, would be wise to keep their air as fresh and clean as possible. Often the only symptoms an owner will notice with an allergic bird is that it may be lethargic and show little interest in its food.

Birds can also develop respiratory allergies, and they may be as sensitive to pollens and mold spores as any other animals. If a bird is kept outside, make sure that the plants surrounding its cage are not highly allergenic. Pollen from early season trees will "prime the pump" and will make the bird more susceptible to allergy later in the year.

The most common allergic reactions in horses are usually urticaria (rash) and chronic obstructive pulmonary disease (COPD). Both of these allergic conditions will be seen most often in stabled horses. Usually these horse allergies are triggered by pollen, or from moldy or dusty hay. Horses with urticaria will often have allergic reactions to bites from gnats, horseflies, mosquitoes, and deerflies. Itching is very common with these types of allergies, and horses will often rub their manes and tails until the hair is thin or gone in these areas.

Horse owners need to be careful about what kind of trees and shrubs they plant around the horse stables and corrals. Leaves and stems of Red Maple (*Acer rubrum*) are poisonous to horses, and these trees should never be planted near corrals or stables. The hay that horses are fed is of the highest quality if it has been cut before it is in full bloom. Late-cut hay will contain much more grass and legume pollen, which may well affect both the horse and its owner.

Hay that was baled when it was not dry enough will get moldy. The spores from this moldy hay are very bad for horses, and they are also bad for people. Dairy farmers often suffer from a condition commonly called "farmer's lung," which is caused by inhaling airborne spores from moldy hay. Although horses are skin tested for allergies by vets and may be given immunology "allergy" shots, the best remedy for a horse with allergies is plenty of fresh, pollen-free hay and dust-free air.

Sheep, goats, and cattle can suffer from allergies, and their symptoms will often be comparable to those experienced by horses. It is worthwhile to note that certain plants that are not poisonous to horses or other mammals may be toxic or allergenic to sheep, goats, or cattle (for example, *Amelanchier alnifolia,* Service Berry). Owners of these animals should have a look at chapter 10, on poisonous plants.

Poisonous Pollen

Poisonous pollen is especially of concern with our pets. It is important to understand that poisonous plants will also have poisonous pollen. If you have pets or small children, please take a look at chapter 10 on poisonous plants and remember that any pollen they have will also be poisonous.

In cold-winter areas, it is fairly common for pets, dogs and cats in particular, to be in direct contact with pollen from male yew (*Taxus* species) shrubs in the landscape. All parts of yews are poisonous, and male yews produce large amounts of pollen in the spring.

In mild-winter areas, close relatives of the yews, *Podocarpus,* are very popular landscape plants. *Podocarpus* (commonly called Yew Pines or Fern Pines) can be spreading ground-cover plants; erect bushy, evergreen shrubs; or even quite large trees. They are all separate sexed, and landscapers prefer to use male plants because they don't shed the messy berries. But male *Podocarpus* will produce huge amounts of pollen each spring that is both allergenic and poisonous. I believe that many pets become seriously ill from pollen of these species and that in most of the cases the cause of the illness is never correctly diagnosed.

How to Diagnose an Animal Allergy

Usually animals will not react the same way to allergens as would a person. With people, sneezing, wheezing, and coughing are the most recognized signs of allergy, but cats that are coughing, wheezing, or that are short of breath are usually thought to be coughing up hair balls. Often what they actually have is feline asthma. Other symptoms of feline asthma are congestion of the sinuses, constant sniffling, or runny noses.

Like cats, dogs also suffer from inhalant allergies from pollens, dust mites, animal dander, and molds. These are all common asthma triggers for people, but dogs usually react differently. Instead of having respiratory symptoms, dogs generally react with skin problems. Constant scratching, biting, chewing, or frequent licking of the feet are also good signs of allergy, as are frequent ear infections. The majority of dogs and cats that are suffering from inhalant allergies never do show any signs of respiratory illness.

Rabbits can get teary eyes or eyes that become matted shut from allergies. Most common allergies of rabbits are caused by pollen and from ammonia fumes. Rabbit cages that are not kept clean will produce ammonia fumes in great amounts. A combination of clean living conditions and plenty of fresh air is the best method for keeping rabbits from developing allergies.

Contact Allergies and Rash-Causing Substances

Be sure to have a look at chapter 9 in this book on plants that can cause skin rashes. Mere contact with the leaves, stems, flowers, or pollen of these plants can sometimes trigger a skin rash in humans or their pets.

A few common animal plant-contact allergies, such as runny eyes from Wandering Jew, or skin conditions from primrose, are well known.

Also of concern, especially with cats, is contact with metals such as nickel, materials like rubber or wool, and chemicals found in dyes and carpet deodorizers, all of which can cause pet allergies.

Dogs or cats can develop allergies to fleabites. Sometimes only one bite can trigger a reaction. Itching is the most common symptom of fleabite allergy.

Sheep and goats can get serious photosensitive skin conditions from eating the big, thick leaves of the common Century Plant, *Agave americana*. *Agave* is not normally considered poisonous, but for sheep and goats if eaten it can trigger not only skin problems but liver problems as well. Bear Grass, also called *Nolina,* is another plant not normally thought of as poisonous, but it will cause sheep and goats skin problems if they eat it.

Allergies from Odors or Fragrances

Hamsters, mice, rabbits, or pet rats often have allergic responses to pet bedding that is made from wood shavings. Shavings from trees such as poplar (aspen) are fine, but often the shavings are made from conifers (cedar, fir, or pine). All of these woods pose special problems for pets. Coniferous wood is usually quite aromatic, and although it may smell good to us, it is important to remember that most animals have much better developed senses of smell than do humans. The smell of the cedar or pine shavings is often so strong that it makes the small rodent pets sick. (More on problems with wood shavings below.) It is important too to note that dogs have an excellent sense of smell and that highly fragrant plants pose more of a threat to them than they do to humans. We may think of fragrances or odors as less substantially problematic since we cannot see them, but fragrance and odors are quite real. They are simply aromatic airborne oils, and with the right camera equipment, these can actually be photographed floating in the air. For some individuals and for many animals, these oils may be just as allergenic as pollen or mold spores.

Cats often develop allergies to the smell of fresh scented kitty litter, especially if the same brand is used over and over again. Cats that are kept inside the house, and dogs too, will also sometimes develop allergies to cigarette smoke, perfumes, cleaners, or to fumes that come from poorly vented furnaces.

Allergies from Wood Shavings

Wood shavings from Western Red Cedar *(Thuja plicata)* contain a powerful insecticide, and the fumes from these shavings may kill small pets; they can also trigger powerful allergic reactions in the person taking care of the pets. The reactions may be immediate, or they may be delayed for many hours, making it difficult to spot the source of the problem. Many people become allergic to dander from caged mice or from the smell of mice, but just as often the allergy is triggered by the cedar shaving bedding used in the mouse cage. Shavings from Eastern Red Cedar *(Thuja occidentalis)* and Japanese Cedar *(Cryptomeria japonica)* contain allergenic properties very similar to those found in Western Red Cedar. (Please note: neither of these species are true cedars, which are in the genus *Cedrus.*) Shavings from pine, although not usually as potent, can sometimes cause severe symptoms. All of these shavings contain natural insecticides that are potentially allergenic.

Studies have found a link between exposure to cedar shavings and oral cancers in both animals and humans. Watch the use of cedar shavings! Sawdust, by the way, from these same trees could be even worse than the shavings as it is much smaller and is more easily inhaled.

Reactions from Eating the Wrong Thing

Dogs are well known to react badly from eating chocolate, and yet many dogs will gladly eat a hunk of chocolate if it's offered. Chocolate is indeed poisonous for dogs, but only in fairly large doses. For example, if your thirty-pound dog grabbed a large Snickers bar and gobbled it down, it wouldn't kill him. If he ate three Snickers bars, though, I'd get him to the vet quick. Unsweetened baking chocolate is by far the most dangerous, while white chocolate has the fewest elements toxic to dogs.

For some reason, as yet not well understood in science, some dogs and cats will get very sick if fed onions, chives, or garlic. Dogs will also get sick from chewing on the common landscape plant Heavenly Bamboo, *Nandina domestica,* even though it is nontoxic to humans. Eating avocados will make many types of birds sick, although it does not affect other types of animals.

Rabbits thrive on good alfalfa and clover hay, but if fed legume hay, rabbits will always have fewer allergies with early cut hay, since alfalfa and clover cut early in the season have less pollen.

Agave is in the Lily family of plants, as are onions, chives, iris, and Daylily. It is worth noting here that plants in this group are not just dangerous to dogs, sheep, and goats, but that Daylily flowers and leaves if eaten are especially toxic to cats.

Food Allergies and Pets

Pets get allergies exactly the same way we do, from constant over-exposure to the same allergen. Almost anything can be a potential allergen, but it is the constant overexposure over time that is needed to develop the allergy. With this in mind, it would be a good idea to vary the food that you feed your pets. Don't feed them the exact same kind of food day in and day out. It is proba-bly boring for the pets as well!

Dogs and cats fed kibble can develop allergies to eggs, whey, milk, preservatives, or most likely to the corn or wheat or other grains that make up most of the kibble. Dogs or cats fed nothing but kibble also can become much more sensitive to related pollens, such as grass pollen. Corn and wheat are, after all, just types of grass. Some people think that expensive pet food is automatically better, but this is not always the case. Allergy can result from any kibble that is fed over and over again.

A dog or cat that develops an allergy to one of the ingredients in kibble can almost always have its health improved by switching to a different diet, one with fewer carbohydrates. Let's take a moment and relate this to us too. If we eat a lot of bread, pasta, rice, or other grain products in the summertime, when grass pollen is abundant, we too will suffer from increased allergies.

Dogs with a food allergy will usually have itchy skin, but many display anal itching, shaking of the head, or ear infections. Food allergies can also cause constant licking of the front paws, rubbing of faces on rugs, and sometimes vomiting, diarrhea, flatulence, sneezing, or asthma-like symptoms. Dogs can occasionally experience behavioral changes from a food allergy, and a friendly dog can even become sullen or aggressive.

Alternative Doggy Diets

If your dog is suffering from allergies, consider switching him or her to a diet primarily of meat, fish, vegetables, and possibly even chicken bones. Dogs fed a diet of mostly meat, vegetables, and bones rarely suffer from allergies. Many people in the United States wouldn't dream of feeding chicken bones to their dog, since of course the dog would choke and die. I used to believe this myself until the day my brother Paul, just returned from living on a kibbutz in Israel, asked me, "Why don't you feed those chicken bones to your dog?"

"Because it would kill him!" I said.

"Well," said my brother, "if that was the case, there wouldn't be a dog left alive in all of Israel. Everyone there feeds chicken bones to their dogs."

I decided to try it and gave my dog, a longhaired Puli named Blackie, some chicken bones. Blackie wolfed down the bones and then quickly started to choke. He spit up the bones and did it all over again. In less than five minutes Blackie had figured out how to eat chicken bones. I've had quite a few dogs since that day and have fed chicken bones to every one of them. I don't advise you do this, but our last dog, a beloved mutt named Sheltie, ate tons of calcium-rich chicken bones, and she lived to be nineteen years old. You should ask your vet for advice on this.

In addition to reducing their allergies, a diet of meats, fish, vegetables, and bones can reduce your dog's weight. Kibble-fed dogs often get too heavy, especially if they don't get lots of exercise. Dogs fed mostly meat and bones will almost never get fat. Diets with excessive carbohydrates are usually the main cause of obesity with both humans and dogs.

Treatment of Animal Allergies

If your animal has obvious allergies, you need to take it to the vet, but you also need to do your part. Much successful treatment with allergies centers on avoidance. Find exactly what your animal is allergic to and then remove that from the animal's environment.

There are other ways to deal with animal allergies that complement allergen avoidance. For example, omega-3 and omega-6 fatty acids are said to be natural anti-inflammatory agents, and many studies conclude that they are useful for dogs that have allergies. Some products for dogs that contain these fatty acids are Omega Pet, Derm Caps, and EFA-Z Plus. Fatty acids, also found naturally in fish oil, are probably good for cats as well, although this is less documented.

Vets do allergy skin testing of cats, dogs, horses, and other animals. They also give immunology shots to many breeds of animals, and often they have fairly good results with these. They also use many different allergy drugs on animals. With cats, vets treat feline asthma and feline allergies with bronchodilators, steroids, and often with antibiotics.

For dog allergies, vets use antihistamines, corticosteroids, and other drugs. Remember, though, that long-term use of steroids can cause numerous problems such as diabetes, decreased resistance to infection, and susceptibility to seizures. Steroids commonly used are drugs such as prednisone, cortisone, and dexamethasone. Steroids, which often are very helpful in alleviating allergy symptoms, must be used in small doses with dogs, and continued long-term usage is dangerous. Cats can often tolerate high doses of steroids, even if dogs cannot.

Dogs are treated with many kinds of antihistamines and seem to tolerate these quite well. Tavist, Benadryl, Chlortrimeton, Atarax, and Seldane are all used successfully for dogs. Apparently the newer drugs such as Allegra and Claritin, which are usually quite effective for people with allergies, do not work as well with dogs. Talk to your vet before dosing your dog with antihistamines.

The most important treatment for pet allergies is eliminating the allergenic triggers. Typical veterinarian medicine, which frequently relies too heavily on use of steroids, is now often being replaced with a more holistic approach. The holistic approach is much more concerned with environmental control, with prevention, with avoidance of the substances that caused the allergies in the first place. Stress always aggravates allergies in animals, and part of a holistic approach always involves ways to limit the individual animal's stress levels. Once you know which substances your animal is allergic to, avoidance is always the best method of control.

Animals and People

New research has shown that children who are raised with several pets are less likely to develop allergies. The explanation behind this is that because these children were exposed to numerous allergens while they were very young, they developed immunities to them. The greatest benefits were found when babies were exposed to pets. Many people try to control allergies with excessive cleanliness, but it appears that just the opposite may well be better for us.

Allergy-Free Animals?

It was reported recently that dark-colored cats are more allergenic for people than light-colored cats, and also that a hypoallergenic cat was being bred. Both of these reports have been met with a good deal of skepticism, but perhaps there's something to them.

There are a few breeds of dogs that are often said to be hypoallergenic. Hard-coated terriers, poodles, and bichon frise are reported to be less likely to cause allergic reactions in susceptible people. I don't know this is true, but it is repeated (by bichon frise and poodle breeders?) often enough that perhaps there may be truth to it. Not only are bichon frise dogs becoming quite popular with allergy sufferers, but so too are Bashkir Curly horses. "Curlies," as they're called, have hair that is more like that of angora than typical horse hair, and some people allergic to horses seem to get along well with their Curlies.

There may be other animals that for one reason or another don't trigger allergies. Some claim Maine coon cats are less allergenic. Apparently Devon rex cats, which have very short, tightly held hair, cause little allergy. These are some unusual-looking cats though! But really, I have my doubts whether or not any of these animals are truly hypoallergenic. In truth, no animal is actually hypoallergic; saliva and urine from any animal may prove to be allergenic. In general longhaired dogs and cats will cause more allergy than will shorthaired ones. I would suggest that you pick up one of these dogs or cats in question, hold him or her for a bit, and see how you feel. As for the allergy-free horses, you could hardly pick up a Curly horse, but I suppose you could take one for a ride.

CHAPTER 12

Stress and Allergies

W hen I was in college I took a class in veterinary science that was given by the head veterinarian of the university, Dr. Dale Smith. Our university was known for its school of agriculture and had a reputation as being a "hands-on" college. As a result we had large herds of cattle, flocks of sheep, pigs, horses, fowl, and so forth.

Dr. Smith had been the university vet for almost thirty years, and his own father had been a vet before him. The first day he told our class, "The most important thing of all for you to be concerned with in animal health is reducing stress. Virtually all the diseases of livestock you will encounter are caused by stress."

He further explained that most genetic diseases had long ago been eliminated with livestock through selective breeding. What you saw instead were animals that were sick because the farmer or rancher wasn't taking care of them properly. They were left outside with no shade in the heat, left with no protection to get out of the wind, stuck in an overcrowded corral, fed a diet too low in nutrients, all of which would cause stress.

"The stress causes a breakdown," said the vet, "and then disease of some kind shows up. It could be a pneumonia, cancer, allergies, any number of things, but stress always sets the stage for this disease."

I have long wondered how it was that a veterinarian understood this so clearly and our own doctors didn't seem to pay much attention to it at all. We are animals after all. Stress must affect us just as it does all the other species of animals. I think most of us who have lived with allergies understand that stress can aggravate the allergies. We'll never be able to eliminate all stress from our lives, but we can learn ways to reduce it, and we can learn ways to deal with it. Whenever possible, it is healthy to try to see some of this stress as a challenge. If we live active lives, we can expect plenty of stress, and that's all right as long as we don't let it get the best of us.

In some ways this whole book is, perhaps more than anything else, about reducing stress. If we don't have the plant in our yard that will cause us a skin rash, then we won't get that rash. If we have female rather than male plants, we won't be inhaling all that pollen and we won't suffer from it. The more allergy-free our yards and gardens are, the less stress there is for us.

But in addition to decreasing the number of allergens, pollen grains, molds, and fungal spores, there are other things we can do to reduce stress in our lives and in our gardens.

Are Allergies Just a Head Trip?

There is a reoccurring problem with stress and allergies. The problem is one of perception. It is well known that stress aggravates allergies. If you did a computer search using the terms "stress, illness, disease," you might be amazed at the hundreds of thousands of entries you'd find. For example, on the website healthdoc.com, there's an article, "Stress, the Number One Cause of Disease and Illness."

Even if the role of stress and illness is not as generally well understood as it ought to be, it is certainly well documented. Stress contributes to heart disease in certain individuals. Stress also contributes to high blood pressure, high cholesterol, and other cardiac risk factors, and many other negative things as well.

Someone with allergies who is under stress will almost certainly experience worse allergies. The problem here is that too many people mix up cause and effect. Allergies are caused by an allergic response to allergens, to perfectly real substances: pollens, molds, dust, dander, allergic plant saps, and so forth.

All too often ignorant people will imply that someone has allergies simply because that person doesn't know how to deal with stress. The implication is that you have allergies because you don't really have your head screwed on straight. This isn't true at all, and actually it is rather insulting. The next step in this illogical progression is that you deserve to have allergies since you're bringing it on yourself. The people making these assumptions are, of course, people who don't have allergies themselves. They don't know how lucky they are, nor do they realize how arrogant are their views. Having persistent allergies can become pretty depressing and frustrating, and critics are often insensitive to this as well.

Yes, allergies can be aggravated by stress, but so can any other illness. Allergies are completely for real. A few examples of this: Years ago when I gave my students different flowers to sniff, we quickly found out that a third of the class reacted strongly to bottlebrush pollen. Later, in blind tests with different types of pollen, the same students all again reacted strongly to the bottlebrush pollen. Another example: I have seen people who were very allergic to shrimp. I have seen what happened to them when they ate some food that they'd been told did not have shrimp in it, but that actually did. They immediately became very ill.

When an allergist skin tests patients, he or she often does the tests on their backs. They can't see the pricks, nor do they know which allergen is being tested with each prick of the skin. Their skin will then react with a welt to the ones they are allergic to. If they are retested soon afterward, the results will be the same. Allergic responses are totally for real, and this simple fact needs to be respected.

Horticultural Stress Reduction

Back to stress. Here are some things we can do to reduce stress in our gardens.

FORGET ABOUT PERFECTION

We don't need perfect gardens, not at all. Our gardens do not need to conform to some ideal. We should have gardens that please us, and that is what's really important. Think of your garden as your place to feel relaxed, to kick back, to unwind. Good gardens can be great stress reducers.

DESIGN

When you first set up your gardens, think about how they will be used. Consider first the function and make them gardens that are a pleasure to be in. If you can possibly afford it, get some professional advice from a landscape designer or a landscape architect. These people are experts on how to create comfortable, attractive, stress-free gardens. In the long run, their advice might turn out to be quite a bargain. With some things you do get what you pay for. With a good designer you get a quality design, one that will long keep you pleased.

While you're thinking about how your landscape might look, buy some of the magazines on landscape design and look them over. See what attracts you. There are some excellent books on landscape design, and these too can help you set up a relaxing, enjoyable garden. I recommend you go down to the bookstore, take some time, and look over all the books on garden design. Even if your yards are already landscaped, these books and magazines are still valuable, because you can always make changes. You can always try to improve your garden.

BIRDS

Wild birds in a garden make it more fun, and just watching them reduces stress. All bird feeders add to your pleasure. I especially love those long, porous mesh bags that you can fill with Niger thistle seed. You hang these over a high branch, and the goldfinches will go crazy for it. Quickly the little goldfinches become almost tame. Just watching them feed is relaxing. The larger, more aggressive sparrows tire quickly of trying to feed from these mesh bags, and this conserves the Niger seed, which as bird seed goes, is a bit pricey.

Hummingbird feeders are great additions to a garden, and who doesn't like to watch hummingbirds? If you can't appreciate hummingbirds, almost certainly your life has far too much stress in it right now. Hang up a hummingbird feeder, relax, and enjoy the show.

A birdbath can be handsome in the garden, and the birds will enjoy it too. Watching robins splash in a birdbath is good karma. Be sure to keep the water clean. A dirty birdbath can spread diseases among the birds, so hosing it out daily is a great idea.

WIND CHIMES

I especially like those bamboo wind chimes, but almost any wind chimes add a nice, mellow touch in the garden. I will admit though that there are a few chimes that are pitched too high for my taste.

The most important thing is that the chimes sound pleasant to you. Hang your chimes in a spot free of obstructions, where they will catch the breeze. When the wind blows, the chimes sing to you.

WATER

Little ponds, tiny waterfalls, water fountains, all of these are proven stress reducers. Certain sounds irritate the human psyche: car alarms blasting in the night, dogs barking on and on. But other sounds, like the sound of splashing water or water tumbling over stones, soothe the soul. Placed in the right spot in a garden, these wet additions can do much for the ambiance of the landscape. Fish in a pond can add quite a bit too. More than one new parent has discovered the calming effect that watching fish swim in an aquarium has on their babies. A few goldfish in a pond are attractive too. A little pond also expands the kinds of plants you can grow in your garden. With a pond you can have water lilies.

Today there are many water fountains available, and some are not too expensive either. Considering their value for reducing stress, they seem like a bargain.

LAWN FURNITURE

This needn't be anything fancy, but every garden ought to have a nice spot or two to sit and relax. A few garden chairs can make a big difference. A little table is good too. Lounge chairs are by design stress busters. When I was young, we had something called a chaise lounge that rocked and was just plain fun to sit in. More stress reduction. If you have an overhanging branch that looks perfect for it, hang a swing from it. Swinging reduces stress too. There has been considerable research into the importance of rocking babies back and forth. Any mother understands how well this works. Perhaps swinging works the same way.

A comfortable garden bench is a worthy addition to any landscape. Place it where two lovers, young or old, can sit and enjoy the view and each other.

READ A BOOK

Seriously, sit in an easy chair in your comfortable garden and read a book. Turn off the TV and go outside. Commune with nature. Read a book on how to reduce stress in your life if you think it might help. Read something on how to maintain a positive, cheery attitude. I find these always give me a boost. But just sitting in the garden and reading a good book is stress reducing. The natural light is good for your eyes and good for all of you. Read a novel if you like. Do sit out in your garden and read. The results are all positive.

FRUIT TREES

Why not use some fruit trees in the landscape? There is something so basic, so fundamentally satisfying to go outside on a warm summer morning and pick a ripe apricot, peach, apple, or plum. Actually, just watching the fruit develop on the tree is satisfying too. If you're inclined and you turn some of that fruit into jams, jellies, pies, or preserves, that's also fantastic. And fruit trees can be perfectly ornamental in the landscape. Few trees look half as good to me as a fruit-laden apricot tree.

If you have the space, consider some kind of a vegetable garden too. There is something about growing tomatoes and string beans that is good for the soul. You certainly don't need a large spot for growing vegetables, although it would be great if you had the room. Working in a vegetable garden is relaxing, something very basic. If you have a spot that gets good sunlight most of the day, consider having some sort of a vegetable garden. Even if it is just a little area where you can grow a few tomato plants each year, the pleasure and stress reduction from this can be incredible.

A BARBECUE

It doesn't need to be elaborate, but if you still enjoy a hamburger or steak or grilled piece of chicken, why not have some kind of a barbecue? Even if you're vegetarian, you can still cook outside on a grill. Bell peppers, chilies, and corn taste great right off a grill. Anyhow, you can get creative. Sometimes this provides a good excuse to sit out in the yard while the food cooks. A barbecue can turn an ordinary meal into a little outdoor adventure.

MOVABLE POTS

I like to have some large pots of flowers that I move around. When they are looking great, I move them up front where everyone can see them. When they are looking ratty, I stick them off on the side of the house to recuperate. I use enough movable pots with enough different kinds of flowers planted in them so I can almost always have something colorful to brighten up any day.

A LAWN

Lawns are supposedly a lot of trouble, but really they are great places for kids to play. Far too many people get hung up on having a "perfect lawn," and with this attitude a lawn can quickly become a big chore. A perfect lawn ought to be a lawn that you like. If it has three different kinds of grasses in it and a dandelion or two and that doesn't bother you, then it's a great lawn. Lawns don't need to be huge; in fact, excessively large lawns are not worth the effort. But a nice small piece of lawn is a people-friendly addition to a garden. If the lawn is a low-pollen type or a pollen-free one, then it's all the better.

PRIVACY

If you like to sunbathe in the nude or just feel like walking out back in your underwear in the morning, you ought to be able to do it without some neighbor looking at you. Front yards can be wide open perhaps, but a backyard needs to provide some privacy. Screens of shrubs or trees can provide this, as can a simple cedar-board fence. Having some privacy in your garden makes it feel like more of a retreat, a spot to get away from the troubles of the world, somewhere to step right out of the rat race. It's a spot for washing away the stresses of everyday life.

CHAPTER 13

Horticultural Therapy and Fen Shui Gardens

The idea of using gardens and plants as "tools" for therapy is growing fast these days. Makes perfect sense too.

The relation between our mental health and our physical health is a close one. Being in positive environments always makes us feel better. If we feel good about ourselves, about our families, our work, our friends, often our bodies will feel stronger too. Just being in a beautiful garden can make us feel better. Doing small chores in the garden – deadheading roses, pulling weeds, planting some bulbs, fertilizing – is good for our physical health too. Fresh air, beauty, some exercise – it's all good for us.

Who's in Charge of Your Garden?

When we talk about the science of gardening, we're talking about horticulture. The more you learn about horticulture, the healthier your gardens can become. One of the things we learn in horticulture is that we are in charge of our gardens. If we don't like the way something is, we can change it.

This is quite unlike the rest of our life. We can't just chop down our boss even if we don't like him or her. We can't just prune away our belly if we suddenly grow alarmed at how large it may have become. Even if our children get on our nerves frequently, we can hardly just uproot them and throw them away.

But in our gardens, in our own landscapes, we are pretty much free to make our own choices. Often when we buy a house, it is already landscaped. It may have a whole hedge of plants we can't stand or a big tree that turns out to be a highly allergenic male clone.

But we are not locked into just putting up with it. Just the opposite! Grant yourself the freedom to do as you please in this area of your life. Experiment all you like in your own yard. If you don't want that shrub or vine or tree, get rid of it and replace it with something you do like. This is one area in which we really are free, and we ought to keep that in mind when we garden.

Attitudes and Gardening

All too often I meet people who act as if their yard is their enemy. They look at their yard, and all they see are things that are not perfect. They tend to think of the garden as a big chore, as a place demanding much work and large expense.

In truth just the opposite can be true. The garden need only be as tidy as you please. You are under no obligation to impress the neighbors. If a dandelion or two pops up in the lawn, you can live with it.

I like beautiful gardens, but there are many kinds of beautiful. Take time to enjoy your garden. Find its beauty. Put a chair or bench here and there, and sit, relax, and admire.

In the Persian language the words "garden" and "heaven" are one and the same. In our own lives so often we spend most of our time rushing here and rushing there. We spend too much time stuck in front of computers, TV sets, stuck in rush-hour traffic, doing things that may be necessary, but things that aren't much fun, much less satisfying.

But working in the garden, that's different, especially for those of us who really do love to garden. I recently saw some research data that suggests that the more tuned into gardening a person is, the more nurturing, creative, and compassionate that person will be. Again, this makes sense. In the garden we are free to experiment. In the garden what we do actually does make a difference, a huge difference. Unlike so many things, the more effort we put into our gardens, the better they are.

What is the link between gardening and empathy for our fellow human beings? Could it be that gardening brings us closer to nature? That by getting in touch with Mother Nature we become more compassionate beings? Probably so. But then too, there's no doubt that the type of people drawn to gardening in the first place may already have in them an extra dose of creativity and compassion.

I used to work in a maximum security prison for juveniles. The CYA it was called, the California Youth Authority. I started the horticulture program there from scratch, and over the years the program grew, the gardens expanded, I learned new things, and so did my wayward students.

Most of my "boys" in the CYA were gang members from the Los Angeles area. Typically they were "in" for armed robbery, muggings, murder. Although they ranged in age from fifteen to twenty-five, most of them could barely read, and none had done any gardening.

I designed our gardens to be therapeutic. We built a big brick barbecue so we could cook things we grew. We grew fruit trees, hundreds of them, so we'd have fresh fruit to eat. We put up bird feeders so we could attract and see birds in the garden. We put up birdbaths, we made wind chimes, and we planted huge gardens of vegetables and flowers.

In our gardens we grew things organically. I taught them to value frogs, toads, lizards, and snakes as welcome additions to the garden. The amphibians and lizards ate many pest bugs, and the snakes ate the equally pesky mice, rats, and gophers. One winter day we adopted a half-frozen kitten, and she became the class cat.

We made huge piles of compost. About the only form of punishment we ever used was "turning the compost heap."

We always had a radio to play some music to listen to while we worked.

Deep, profound changes happened to many of these hardened criminals while working in the garden. As they learned to hybridize roses, they lost their desire to rob liquor stores. As they grew tomatoes big as your fist and watermelons big as beach balls, they became proud of their accomplishments. The more they learned about plants, the less they were interested in crime.

Many of these boys learned how to read, to do math, to write, and learned it all there in the gardens, in the greenhouses. When I taught math, all the examples dealt with square footage of gardens, pounds of fertilizer to be applied, or perhaps cubic yards of mulch to buy for landscape jobs. I would often have a student follow me and read to me from a book as I walked around supervising the work in the gardens.

I worked in the CYA for twelve years. People in authority sometimes claimed that I bribed my "wards" and that I must be doing something illegal. They couldn't understand how it was that these guys could learn the scientific names of hundreds of plants and that they actually learned to love to read, to love to garden. Most of the people in charge felt that these wards of ours would never amount to anything, that they were beyond repair. But I didn't bribe the boys, I just set up a garden with a healing atmosphere and then let it work its wonders.

A good garden can be a magical place. Let me explain. Plants are not judgmental. You take good care of them, and they thrive. In the garden our minds are free to wander, to daydream, to relax. Good things happen in good gardens.

Why talk about horticultural therapy in a book devoted largely to allergy avoidance? The answer is simple. Gardening itself can be very therapeutic – whether it helps keep you in shape, abandon crime, or just be more relaxed. However, if the garden is filled with plants that cause allergies, the gardening experience won't be that good. It's no fun to be sneezing and even less fun to have attacks of skin rashes or asthma. By making our gardens allergy-free we can avoid these negatives. The physical work done in gardens is also good for us, burning calories, making our muscles stronger. In the right garden the air is cleaner, too, refreshing our lungs as we work.

It just makes sense to have a therapeutic garden be allergy-free. Ultimately *Safe Sex in the Garden* is about being healthy.

The Fen Shui Garden

The more people you talk to about fen shui and gardening, the more opinions on it you get. A landscape designer once told me, "Fen shui gardening is really just good landscape design."

And to a point, I would agree with her. In many ways the ancient Chinese philosophy of fen shui, also called feng shui, is all about creating harmony. In a true fen shui garden the focus is on the atmosphere. A garden is created that encourages meditation, relaxation, and close connections to nature.

A good fen shui garden does not ignore any of our senses. There are fragrant flowers to smell, wind chimes, the sounds of water, the songs of birds to please our ears, shade from the hot sun, protection from the wind, places just to sit and think, contrasting surfaces to feel, beauty to please our eye, and perhaps even some fruit or vegetable for our tongue to taste.

A true fen shui garden is not strictly formal, overly clipped, too tidy and sanitary, all drawn with squares and rectangles. Shrubs don't need to be square nor do all trees need to resemble each other. A quiet restrained informality is encouraged. Love, peace, understanding, and wisdom reign in a true fen shui garden.

In many ways during all my years at the Youth Authority, although I didn't know it at the time, I was instinctively trying to develop a fen shui garden. Surrounded by guards, gangs, and concertina razor wire, I aspired to create an inner sanctum, a natural place for me and my students to remove ourselves from all the bad vibes so very close by.

I am not a fen shui expert by any means, but I have read a great deal about it, have listened to numerous talks by experts, and I have long been interested and involved in garden design. I think that fen shui does indeed have much to offer and that it is well worth exploring. Unfortunately I often notice a certain snobbishness surrounding the subject. One expert writes that none of the others know what they're talking about, especially the Western writers and speakers. I've met some fen shui designers and writers who were cold and impersonal, none of which jives with true fen shui in my mind.

My feeling about attitudes in gardening – fen shui or otherwise – is this: Elitism doesn't belong in the garden. Plants aren't critical; let's not be that way ourselves. Many people, far wiser than I, have long known that the more we learn about something, the more we realize how little we know. Harold Young, the wonderful senior editor of *Pacific Coast Nurseryman* magazine, once wrote me in an email, "I used to think I knew a lot of plants."

I know just what he means. Horticulture is a huge subject, and no matter how experienced we are, none of us will ever know the half of it. So let's not be too snobby or critical. Let's just create healthy, allergy-free gardens that are pleasing to us – however fen shui or not they may be.

CHAPTER 14

Going Organic—
How to Get Started

I have an M.S. in agriculture, and back when I was a college student I used to take a lot of heat from my professors because I was interested in organic farming and organic gardening. In the 1960s to be in agriculture and to be interested in organic gardening was to automatically be labeled as one of those dreaded "hippies." But many organic methods always made plenty of sense, and some can save considerable amounts of money. These days even commercial agriculture is coming around to organic methods, if slowly. Today the newest buzzword in agricultural universities is "sustainable agriculture," and I'm all for it. But honestly, much of sustainable agriculture is simply rediscovered, reformulated organic gardening. So far I have resisted the urge to say, "Hey, I told you so!"

Why go organic? Isn't it an awful lot of trouble? Yes, it is some trouble, and it certainly isn't always the fastest way or the most "efficient" way to garden, but it's worth it. Let me explain.

Side Effects of Common Garden Chemicals

Much has been written about the dangers from chemical garden bug killers, and much of this bears repeating – especially here in a book about the interactions among people, plants, and human health.

Most of us have a tendency not to take too seriously things we can't see, and sometimes this is a bad mistake. Just because something is microscopic doesn't mean it can't affect us.

Almost everyone who can read knows now about the terrible aftereffects of all that DDT used with the advent of the "chemical revolution." But what of the so-called safe garden chemicals we are so often encouraged to use? Just how safe are they?

For anyone who hasn't yet read the masterpiece *Silent Spring* by Rachel Carson, I suggest you do. If you read it years ago as I did, you might want to read it again. Rachel Carson was the biologist who uncovered incredible damage to the environment from pesticides. Carson basically blew the whistle on the chemical companies, and her work has had a hugely beneficial impact on the environment. Nonetheless, you'd probably be surprised at how much was known back in the early 1960s and how much of that information has to this very day been ignored.

A recent article in the *Los Angeles Times* entitled "Centers for Disease Control to Detail Blood Contaminants" was quite alarming. Blood from a representative five thousand Americans was tested for chemicals, and some surprising, alarming things were found.[1]

Such garden-variety pesticides as Malathion and diazinon are supposedly relatively harmless since they break down so quickly in the body. But this newest study found that "higher-than-expected levels" of these chemicals were found in the sampled blood.

What does this mean? I would interpret this to mean that (1) these chemicals don't break down in our bodies as quickly as claimed, or (2) there is so much of this poison being sprayed on almost everything we eat that we are constantly being reexposed to it, or (3) perhaps a combination of both 1 and 2 are at work.

What was the chemical industry's reaction to this? The American Chemistry Council's "public health team" spokesperson said, "It [the CDC finding] is virtually impossible to interpret."

I don't think so! Do you? I think the findings are perfectly clear and are easily interpreted. It seems to me that the chemical companies did not want to correctly interpret this data. To do so honestly would be paramount to admitting fault. To date no chemical companies have been big on ever admitting fault. (As a parallel it might be worth noting that to date the tobacco companies have never admitted that cigarettes are unhealthy, much less that they can cause cancer.) Simply, the chemical pesticides we have long been told were perfectly safe are not. They are turning up in our blood at rates higher than expected, and they obviously do not break down as quickly in our bodies as we have been led to believe.

Poisons Are Poison — Break the Habit

Many of us, myself included, used to think we had to spray a certain amount of these pesticides, certainly on our fruit trees. My parents have an old apple tree that my dad used to spray every year, numerous times, with sevin, Malathion, and dormant sprays. Every year he still always got a certain amount of codling moth worms in some of the apples no matter how much he sprayed.

Six years ago I talked him into stopping this spraying. Now he still has some apples that get the worms, but at least he isn't spraying. Does he have more wormy apples than he used to? Perhaps. But really there isn't a noticeable difference. And most of the somewhat wormy apples can still be cut up for good applesauce – organic applesauce.

Allergy and Pesticides

Applying pesticides is often far from a precise science. When we are spraying pesticides with a pump or power sprayer, it is very easy to get some of this material on us, especially if there is any breeze. In the trade they call this contamination "drift." Many of you know all about this and have experienced this drift yourself when the wind suddenly changed, or when you tried to get the spray on a particularly high branch.

Based on the newest CDC findings drift is dangerous, but it would appear that even without drift, use of these garden chemicals is dangerous. For anyone with allergies, it is doubly so. Frequently people who have had as few as one or two heavy exposures to chemical pesticides have a severe breakdown of their immune systems. Some people who never had allergies before suddenly become allergic to a great many things.

I suggest you give up chemical pesticides. Don't worry, the great chemical companies won't go out of business. But you'll save some money, and in the long run you may save your health too. Your plants will be just fine too, maybe even better.

How "Pure" Do I Have to Be?

Really, you don't "have" to take any of these suggestions. But since you asked, why not break as many of these chemical habits as you can? Any chemicals you quit using in your garden can be a plus. If you simply must use your chemical fungicide on your hybrid tea roses, so be it. But use plenty of caution with it. If you just have to use dandelion killer on your perfect fescue sod lawn, go for it, but don't track that stuff in the house. This isn't a perfect world, and I know that not everyone is willing to go whole hog organic, but be a sport, do as much as you can.

Why not have your whole garden, including your soil, be as organic as possible? Good dirt is the foundation of all fine gardens, and with soil, the more humus (organic matter) the better. Start a compost heap or an earthworm pit, and use that vegetable garbage instead of tossing it in the trash. Don't toss those coffee grounds – add them to your compost heap.

Mulch your flowerbeds instead of raking them "clean" down to the bare ground. Use those old leaves instead of bagging and tossing them.

Organic Spraying

Here's the fun part – we don't have to give up spraying. We just have to change the way we do it and the ingredients we use.

The simplest safe insecticide is made of dish soap, water, and vegetable oil. I mix 2 to 4 tablespoons of soap with 2 tablespoons of any kind of vegetable oil, in a gallon of warm water. Used often enough, this mix will kill all insect pests. I use this mix frequently. (There are other simple and safe methods of pest control, covered in more detail in chapter 8.) Will these less toxic methods be "every bit as effective as the most powerful chemical sprays"? Nope. They won't be. Sometimes you may have to repeat them five or six times to get the effect you're looking for, but they are safer – and less expensive too.

Some Good Sources for Help

Take a look at the sections at the end of this book on helpful websites and recommended books. Get the best advice on organic fertilizers, organic pest control, organic lawn care, organic fruit and vegetable gardening. Lots of good advice there on going organic.

CHAPTER 15

CO_2, Global Warming, and Pollen Allergies

The benefits of adding organic matter to the soil have long been known. These benefits usually include increased nitrogen, greater water-holding capacity, and an increase in activity of soil earthworms and microbes. Experiments have shown that the increase in carbon dioxide (CO_2) release that accompanies added organic matter is certainly one of the main reasons why adding organic matter to the soil increases plant growth.

Greenhouse owners have long understood that plants consume CO_2 and release oxygen. In a greenhouse packed full of plants, the plants, through the process of photosynthesis, can quickly use up most of the available CO_2. Then their growth slows down or stops. To compensate for this, old-time growers used to place boxes or flats of fresh manure underneath their greenhouse benches. As the manure decomposed it released CO_2 into the greenhouse air, and the plants grew faster as a result.

In today's modern greenhouses, especially those with concrete floors, lack of CO_2 is always a concern. (Concrete keeps CO_2 from coming up from the soil.) Most of the newer greenhouse ranges are now equipped with automatic CO_2 regulators that monitor the amount of CO_2 in the air inside the greenhouse and then release more as needed. In these greenhouses with their gas growth CO_2 generators, the plants don't just grow bigger, they also mature earlier.

So what has all this to do with global warming and allergies? As we become more and more reliant on burning petroleum products and as our global temperatures continue to rise, carbon dioxide levels in our air are rising. Before the last election we in the United States had assumed, incorrectly, that no matter which candidate won the election, new controls were going to be placed on CO_2 emissions.

We know better now.

The United States, with its huge consumption of fossil fuels (the United States produces nearly 25 percent of man-made carbon dioxide emissions worldwide), is also experiencing the greatest increase in CO_2. Actually CO_2 accounts for 80 to 85 percent of the heat trapping (greenhouse) gases contributing to global warming.

The idea that is now called the "greening theory" holds that all this extra CO_2 is good. It will result in increased plant growth and thus in resulting increases in food supplies. There is some merit to this theory, but there are numerous downsides too.

Pollen Allergies

There are many negative effects from global warming – polar ice cap melt, more smog, flooded low-lying islands, disappearance of certain native species, etc. – but let's just consider one here: pollen production and its effect on allergies.

Since 1959 allergies have dramatically increased in the United States, from 2 to 5 percent of the population affected to a whopping 38 percent now.

Largely because of the huge horticultural "success" of the much oversimplified theory of "litter-free" landscaping, we already have vast urban landscapes that are heavily loaded with wind-pollinated dioecious male cultivars (clones) of trees and shrubs. These modern landscape trees fill the surrounding air with unnaturally large amounts of allergenic pollen. Because the "messy" urban female trees are now so rare, almost none of this pollen is now trapped, removed from the air, and turned into seed. (Female trees produce no pollen, ever, but they do make seeds, pods, and fruit.)

We have tidy sidewalks but pollen-filled air.

Under normal carbon dioxide levels, these male cloned trees will always produce abundant amounts of pollen. Under increased levels of carbon dioxide, they produce considerably more. The increase in temperature itself (just one effect of too much greenhouse gas in the air) also results in increased pollen production as well as in pollen production that starts earlier in the spring and lasts further into the fall.

Research shows that under stress conditions male plants are able to take up more water than are females. Under stress conditions, such as drought, male trees are also able to hold onto the water they already have better than are female trees. This is like adding insult to injury, since it means that our scarce urban female trees are more likely to die early from stress than are the numerous allergy-causing male trees.

Where there are abundant water and soil nutrient sources, the increases in carbon dioxide levels in our air will result in larger urban trees, which, if they're allergy trees, will be capable of producing ever more pollen.

Increases in carbon dioxide increase plant growth, but only if there is enough available water and nitrogen in the soil to support this additional growth. When the supplies of water and nutrients are not adequate to support this added CO_2-induced growth, interesting physiological things happen in plants. Foremost, it is an added stress on the plants, and stress often results in an increase in unusual reproduction factors.

A stressed lemon tree, for example, will often produce a huge crop of tiny, very seedy lemons. This is simply the lemon tree's way of preparing for its own imminent demise and also for its own legacy of possible seedlings.

Another stress example: In daily pollen collections taken by biology professor Dr. Lee Parker and his students from the top of the Fisher Science Building at California Polytechnic State University (Cal Poly), San Luis Obispo, during the middle of a severe seven-year drought, all-time record oak pollen levels were recorded. The severely drought-stressed oaks were responding to their possible premature demise – by overproduction of the tree's chief male sexual expression, pollen.

Stress also makes tree species mature earlier than normal. With urban landscapes, this can bring yet more allergy. In the past twenty years in particular there has been a huge increase in this planting of male-cloned street trees, but these trees cannot produce pollen until they mature. With the increases in CO_2 levels, we can predict that they will mature earlier than expected.

University and United States Department of Agriculture (USDA) researchers have recently found some alarming connections between global warming and pollen production.

Shannon L. LaDeau and J. S. Clark, researchers at Duke University, found that pine trees grown with elevated levels of CO_2 produced three times the normal amount of seeds and also matured prematurely.[1]

Lewis H. Ziska, Ph.D., a USDA researcher, recently found that increased CO_2 resulted in huge increases in the pollen production of ragweed and other weeds.[2]

Nancy Tuchman, a biology professor at Loyola University in Chicago, is also researching the feed value of CO_2-enhanced leaves on microorganisms and insects. She found that they all grow slower when fed these "enhanced" leaves. "If all the plants are altered on a global level, then it's certainly going to affect all the organisms on Earth," she said. "No one is going to escape."[3]

Compounding all of this is that excessive burning of fossil fuels and the resulting pollution may well be compromising our very endocrine and immune systems. Theo Colburn explored this well in the very interesting book *Our Stolen Future* (Penguin Books, 1996).

Great increases in the already excessively high rates of urban pollen, combined with further compromised immune systems, may well be the recipe for allergies of true epidemic proportions in the not too distant future.

Dr. Robert C. Stebbins, renowned biologist from the University of California at Berkeley, and author of the fabulous *Western Field Guide to Reptiles and Amphibians,* told me recently in a phone conversation that the planting of all these male dioecious and altered monoecious trees "is a classic example of how they just didn't think about the ecology involved."

Unfortunately politics plays a big part in the debate about global warming. Auto companies insist on churning out an ever-growing supply of gas-guzzling SUVs. Consumers insist on their right to drive their 4WD monster trucks. Certain politicians insist on their constituents' rights as Americans to own these enormous gas hogs. Nonetheless, if we don't start paying closer attention to how we landscape our cities, and we don't start getting serious about better gas mileage and alternative clean energy sources, rampant allergies may well be the end result. It could be a gold mine for pharmaceutical corporations, but it will be a nightmare for the rest of us.

CHAPTER 16

Smog Trees and Super-Trees

In this chapter let's explore the subject of the smog-forming gases that are released by some of our trees. At the same time I want to identify the ones that cause the most problems and also the ones that have just the opposite effect.

VOCs: Volatile Organic Compounds

In *Allergy-Free Gardening* I called the subject of plant-produced volatile organic compounds (VOCs) "horticulture's dirty little secret." Some species of plants produce huge amounts of these smog components, and the fact that they do has been under study for more than thirty years now. But it has long been extremely unpopular to say or write anything negative about plants and about trees in particular. Why is this?

For starters some very beloved trees, like many species of oak, happen to fall into the high-VOC category. This just doesn't sit well with some folks. There are large civic tree organizations that promote the idea that all trees are wonderful, and they are in no rush to promote this material. Huge sums of money are tied up in many of these species in the nursery industry, and no business likes to lose money. It's not been a popular subject by any means!

Not all plants are of the same value to us. Is a poison ivy vine as valuable to society as an apple tree? Is ragweed as important to us as corn? No doubt these noxious plants have their place in the wild, but not in the city. I did actually recently hear a fellow claim proudly that he had planted poison ivy on his land, since it was native. It made sense to him, but it doesn't to me, native or not.

Many trees, otherwise wonderful, are not healthy additions in urban settings. Largely because of smog and diesel fumes, people living in cities are more susceptible to allergies, and it is important that we stop planting high-allergy trees inside the city limits. Likewise, in the city we are much more affected by smog components, and we need to consider this with every city tree we plant.

So What Exactly Are VOCs?

Organic chemicals are found in all living things or in products (such as lumber, oil, or coal) that once were living things. Some organic chemicals never occur in nature but have been synthesized by chemists. The common high-nitrogen, synthetic fertilizer urea is a good example. It is "organic" but not "natural."

An organic compound contains carbon and hydrogen. Sugar (which contains carbon, hydrogen, and oxygen), for example, is an organic compound, but it is not volatile. Volatile chemicals produce vapors that can easily escape into the air. Volatile organic chemicals include industrial chemicals such as benzene, solvents such as toluene and xylene, and gasoline. Many volatile organic chemicals are especially hazardous air pollutants.

Organic compounds that evaporate easily are called volatile organic compounds – VOCs. Some common health effects from overexposure to VOCs are headaches, irritated eyes, sinus conditions, breathing problems, dizziness, and nausea.

Smog

The two main VOCs produced by plants are ozone (O_3) and carbon monoxide (CO). When combined with sunlight and the chief air pollutant from petroleum-burning engines, NOx (nitrogen oxide compounds), the end product, in layperson's terms, is smog. VOCs are produced in other ways too – from volcanoes and forest fires. VOCs that are released by plants are also called "biogenic emissions."

When we speak of ozone here, we are talking about ground-level tropospheric ozone, the main smog ingredient that irritates our eyes and lungs on smoggy days. This type of ozone is a heat-trapping, colorless greenhouse gas that contributes to global warming and is especially hazardous to young children and the elderly. It seems the very young and the very old are always the ones at most risk for so many ill things, be it ozone, pneumonia, or West Nile virus. Tropospheric ozone can also aggravate asthma and cause breathing problems, even in healthy adults. This ground-level ozone is of particular concern on hot, humid summer days.

There is another type of ozone, stratospheric ozone, which is the protective ozone. This is the ozone that, ten to thirty miles up in the atmosphere, absorbs ultraviolet radiation and protects our skin from the direct rays of sunlight. When people write or talk about the "hole in the ozone," they are talking about this stratospheric ozone. This is not the same ozone we refer to when discussing plant-produced VOCs. However, to be perfectly honest here, ozone is ozone, and tropospheric and stratospheric ozone are the same thing. It is just that when ozone is far up in the atmosphere, it is protective, and when it is down close to ground level, it is a pollutant.

CO, carbon monoxide, is the other main pollutant of tree VOCs. CO is colorless, odorless, and extremely toxic. CO is the most deadly ingredient of smoke. Diesel exhaust from trucks and fumes from heaters may have large amounts of CO in them. CO is combustible, often hard to detect, and has been implicated directly or indirectly in deaths from many causes. CO aggravates allergies, and asthma. CO poisoning is thought to sometimes be a factor in sudden infant death syndrome (SIDS).

Horticulture and VOCs

All right, so what does this have to do with gardening and horticulture? Quite a bit, actually! VOCs are a major component of smog. We all know what smog is – that dirty, irritating, eye-burning haze that has replaced blue sky in far too many modern cities today. Does smog cause allergies? We don't know for sure, but we do know that it certainly aggravates allergies. Smog makes it harder to breathe in the first place and clogs up our airways, making them more susceptible to allergens like pollen or mold spores. Many researchers now believe that certain types of smog actually cause allergies.

Fortunately, all is not lost: Some species of plants release large amounts of VOCs, and other species remove them. In some areas more VOCs are produced by the area's trees than by human activities!

Whoa! This sounds like trash journalism, but it's true. Back in the late 1960s, California's then governor, Ronald Reagan, said in a speech that trees were causing smog. He was quickly ridiculed for this stance and just as quickly backed away from it. But – as much as some of us might hate to admit he was right, on this he was certainly at least partially correct.

It is of course possible that the governor brought up the issue of smog-producing trees as an excuse not to worry so much about other forms of pollution. What really blows my mind, though, is that all these years later this entire business about VOC-producing trees has remained buried so deep. Everyone claims to be concerned about pollution and smog, but so far few have done anything about natural pollution. Again, it is not a popular topic, and it is not politically correct to blame nature for anything. However, city landscapes are not exactly unadulterated nature by any means.

However, we are now finally starting to see some material on plant-produced VOCs coming to the surface. Urban foresters are now starting to take note, and hopefully attention to this will only increase.

How Dangerous Is Smog?

When you are at a certain altitude and can look down on a city cloaked in its filthy cover of smog, does it look healthy to you? Of course not, and it isn't healthy in the least. Back in 1984 a study conducted by Dr. Kay Kilburn, M.D., Professor of Medicine at the University of Southern California, found that children raised in the smoggy Los Angeles South Coast Air Basin suffered a 10 to 15 percent decrease in lung function compared with children who grew up where the air was less polluted.

Children's lungs are not fully developed, which leaves them more susceptible to harm from smog. Because many children are very active, they may have far more air exchanges (breathing in and breathing out) per day than would a more sedentary adult. Because of the high number of air exchanges with children (and with all endurance athletes too), they are considerably more at risk from all airborne pollutants, be they smog, dust, spores, or pollen.

There are a huge number of interesting studies on the negative health effects of smog. For example, David Abbey, Ph.D., of Loma Linda University (Loma Linda, California), studied a group of 6,340 Seventh Day Adventists living throughout California (62 percent lived in the smoggy Los Angeles Basin). Results of his study suggest a strong relationship between long-term exposure to air pollution and development of certain chronic diseases. People living in high-smog areas had higher risks of respiratory diseases, including a 33 percent greater bronchitis risk and 74 percent greater asthma risk. In addition, women living in the smoggiest areas had a 37 percent higher risk of developing some form of cancer. Smog should not be taken lightly and certainly ought not to just be accepted.

If we who plant trees can do something about it, we ought to get to it. So what can we do?

It is important to understand that all trees that are low VOC emitters are, unfortunately, not necessarily low-allergy trees. Neither are all allergy-friendly, pollen-free trees necessarily low-VOC emitting trees. For example, a female beefwood tree, *Casuarina stricta*, is a pollen-free tree that will help to remove allergenic ambient *Casuarina* pollen (from male beefwood trees) from the air. Nonetheless, all beefwoods are high VOC-emitting trees, so even this easy-on-your-allergies tree could still contribute to smog formation. My suggestion, therefore, is to use mainly low VOC-emitting female trees in the city. In the countryside, where there is much less (human made) NOx in the air, use any female tree or shrub you like. Remember, in order for tree emissions to become smog, they must first combine with NOx.

Smog Trees, Allergy Trees, and Super-Trees

Smog trees are those trees that emit very high amounts of VOCs and remove very little. Allergy trees are those trees that produce large amounts of highly allergenic pollen. Super-Trees are trees that are net VOC consumers and are also pollen-free. Here are several suggestions for cleaner city air:

- Plant very few street trees, if any, that produce large amounts of VOCs.

- Plant very few, if any, street trees that produce large amounts of allergenic pollen.

- Do not plant any more urban trees that combine large output of allergenic pollen and VOCs! Some examples of these are male willows, male poplars, most *Eucalyptus,* most species of oaks, male *Casuarina* (beefwood), and male Sour Gum (*Nyssa* species) trees.

- Do plant millions of those wonderful trees that consume more VOCs than they produce *and* that also do not produce allergenic pollen. *Do* plant millions of these Super-Trees! When we can combine the best of both, it's a win-win situation for everyone. A list of Super-Trees follows this section (after a list of the VOC "dirty dozen").

- While we're at it, let's plant as many other kinds of plants as we can – grasses, shrubs, and flowers – that combine the allergy *and* smog-fighting qualities of the Super-Trees. Some examples are female junipers, female yews, disease-resistant roses, and female Buffalo Grass.

- Whenever possible, plant deciduous Super-Trees that will mature at a large size. The larger they grow, the more shade they will provide in summer, cutting cooling costs. The larger they grow the more VOCs, dust, and pollen they will remove. The larger these Super-Trees grow, the more oxygen they will pump into our towns. Shade from these big Super-Trees will cool the area around them, resulting in less smog because fewer VOCs are produced when it is cooler. The rate of VOC emissions from plants is not constant. It increases with hot weather and decreases with cool conditions.

- There are other advantages to large urban deciduous trees. They lose their leaves in winter and let in the warming winter sun, resulting in lower heating costs and lower fossil fuel emissions. Large urban trees also provide needed habitat for animals, birds, and beneficial insects. These big trees help to absorb much of the noise of the city. Big Super-Trees don't just add material physical health blessings to their surroundings; their very presence provides a soothing, pleasing counterbalance to the stress of everyday city life.

- Large evergreen Super-Trees can be well used where they will act as windbreaks and where they will not cast unwanted shade in winter. In the right place in the landscape, these are extremely valuable trees. When we plant tall evergreen trees or hedges that will grow tall, however, we need to take into consideration how they will eventually affect our neighbors living closest to them. A tall evergreen hedge on the west side of your house may cut off the entire wonderful, warm, early morning eastern sunlight for your neighbor who is just west of you.

- Let's start driving cars that get decent mileage. I have an old 1988 Mazda 626 with 237,000 miles on it (same engine, same clutch) that still gets over forty miles per gallon on the highway. The less gas we burn, the less NOx we pump into the air. Let's not wait for the government to do something. Let's get into driving cars that get good mileage. We'll save some money while we do our part for cleaner air.

- Let's have more light-colored roofs, light-colored buildings, and light-colored pavement and streets, especially in our southern areas. Light- rather than dark-colored streets and buildings will reflect hot sunlight, keep us cooler, and will reduce VOC production. Urban areas are often much warmer than their surrounding areas. This is because the city roads and buildings absorb so much heat. The more heat, the more VOCs that are released.

The plants listed below all produce more VOCs than they consume. It is important to understand that some VOC-emitting species are much worse than others. For example, a Gambel Oak may produce ten times more VOCs than a spruce.

THE VOC DIRTY DOZEN

Listed on a 1 to 12 basis, where 12 is the most VOC emitting:

1. Spruce
2. Black Gum *(Nyssa)*
3. Willow
4. Aspen
5. Acacia
6. Black Locust *(Robinia)*
7. Carrotwood trees *(Cupaniopsis)*
8. Sycamore
9. Eucalyptus
10. Beefwood *(Casuarina)*
11. Sweet Gum
12. Gambel Oak

And here's a list of the very opposite sort of plants, best suited for cleaning air in our cities. The trees and shrubs listed below are all net VOC removers. These are some common landscape plants that remove carbon monoxide and ozone from the air. This list is by no means complete, but these are some good ones.

Apricot trees

Ash trees (female ash trees are allergy free)

Avocado trees

Basswood or linden trees

Box Elder trees (see Maple trees below; female Box Elders are also pollen free)

Buckeye trees

Cedar trees (female trees are allergy free)

Cherry trees

Chinese Scholar Tree

Chinese Tulip Poplar

Dogwood trees and shrubs

Fringe Trees (females are pollen free)

Hawthorn trees and shrubs

Holly trees and shrubs (female hollies are allergy free)

Honey Locust trees (females would be allergy free)

Hydrangea

Juniper trees and shrubs (females are allergy free)

Loquat trees

Maple trees (female trees are allergy free)

Mountain ash (*Sorbus* species)

Mulberry trees (female trees are allergy free)

Nectarine trees

Orange trees

Osmanthus trees and shrubs

Paulownia trees

Peach trees

Pear trees

Persimmon

Plum trees

Pomegranate

Redbud trees

Sourwood trees *(Oxydendrom)*

Strawberry Tree *(Arbutus unedo)*

Tree-of-Heaven (*Ailanthus* female trees are pollen free)

Viburnum trees and shrubs

Existing Trees in the Landscape

For trees that are already well established and growing well, consideration of their total societal value should always include the sex of the tree if they are separate-sexed (dioecious). Also very important is whether or not they are of a species that is known to be a net producer or net remover of VOCs. City tree committees, for example, should almost never approve the removal of a healthy female tree that is both pollen free and known to be of a net VOC-removing species.

Some Super-Trees

In all circumstances, the chosen tree must be one that is well adapted to the area where it is to be planted. This will help insure that it will thrive and not become an insect-infested tree that produces abundant insect dander and mold spores. Plant zones, for those not familiar with them, are geographical areas where certain plants will or will not grow. There are different zone schemes, but the one I use is the simple, old, long-used USDA 1 to 10 zone map. With this system, zone 1 has the coldest, harshest winters, and zone 10 is warm, usually southern and coastal, and always mild wintered. Frost is rare in zones 9 and 10, even in the middle of winter.

A zone 2 plant will almost always fail to thrive if planted in, say, zone 10. Likewise a zone 8 plant will fail to thrive if planted in zone 7. A zone 8 plant that is planted in zones 1–6 would probably be winter killed the very first winter.

The following are some highly recommended Super-Trees. This list is by no means exhaustive; there are other fine Super-Trees to be had. Again, a Super-Tree is any tree that is net VOC-consuming AND one that is also a pollen-free or very low-pollen producing tree.

Ash trees, _Fraxinus_ species, are separate sexed and remove VOCs. Two quite similar ash cultivars that are all female are ***Fraxinus angustifolia* 'Flame'** and *F. angustifolia* **'Moraine.'** These are winter hardy, easy to grow, easy to find, large-growing Super-Trees. Winter hardy zones 3–10.

There are several other ash cultivars that would also qualify as Super-Trees. *Fraxinus excelsior* **'Pendula'** is an interesting example. Called the Weeping English Ash, it must be grafted on an ash seedling since it is entirely weeping in form, much like the Weeping Mulberry tree. Also, like the Weeping Mulberry, the Weeping English Ash is pollen free and consumes VOCs. Winter hardy zones 5–10.

'Summit' Ash (*Fraxinus pennsylvanica* **'Summit'**) is a very large, common, widely adapted, quite winter-hardy tree that, although female, does not produce many seeds. 'Summit' is a very useful big Super-Tree. Winter hardy zones 3–10.

'Tomlinson' ash (*Fraxinus uhdei* **'Tomlinson'**) is an excellent ash tree for mild-winter areas. 'Tomlinson' is thought to be a hybrid, and besides having thick, attractive leaves, it also apparently never flowers at all. This would not make it very useful for trapping ash pollen, but nonetheless it is a pollen-free tree itself. Growing to almost eighty feet tall under good conditions, 'Tomlinson' has qualities to please almost everyone: pollen free, VOC consuming, and litter free. Winter hardy in zones 5–10.

Box Elder 'Variegatum' *(Acer negundo* **'Variegatum')** is female, deciduous, has attractive variegated leaves, is easy to find in nurseries, is extra winter-hardy and widely adapted, and is exceptionally good at attracting the most allergenic types of pollen. The variegated Box Elder is also remarkably productive at removing VOCs from the air. Winter hardy in zones 3–10.

Cedar trees (*Cedrus* species): *Cedrus atlantica* (the Atlas Cedar), *Cedrus brevifolia* (the Cypress Cedar), *Cedrus Deodara* (the Deodar Cedar), and *Cedrus libani* (the Cedar of Lebanon). These are all true cedars. All are evergreen coniferous trees, related to pines. They are usually separate sexed. Cedar cones always point straight up on the branches. Male cones on male trees are far more numerous than female cones on female trees. Female cones, which look almost like wooden roses when matured and open, are much larger in size than male cones. Only female cedars are Super-Trees.

Cedar trees are excellent net VOC removers, and the female trees with their fat upright cones (prior to maturity) are pollen free. Any female true cedar is therefore a Super-Tree. Please note: There are many trees and shrubs that are commonly called "cedars" that are usually anything but. Cedars have short, stiff needlelike evergreen leaves and cones that grow upright. There are only four species of true cedars—the four listed above. Winter hardy in zones 6–10.

***Ilex* species, the hollies,** are all separate sexed, and all of them are also excellent VOC removers. Essentially this means that any large, tall-growing holly that is female is a Super-Tree. Female hollies are easy to recognize since they're the ones with the red berries. Deciduous hollies are more winter hardy than the evergreen species. Hardiness varies considerably from species to species, but there are some hardy species of holly that can be grown in zones 3–4, and many species that are hardy in zones 5–10.

While all female junipers are pollen free, male junipers are anything but. Male junipers, which are extremely common landscape shrubs and trees, produce huge amounts of allergenic pollen.

Juniperus chinensis 'Torulosa,' the Hollywood Juniper, is also called the Twisted Juniper. This is one of the most common large junipers used in mild-winter areas. Lucky for us it is one that is pollen free and consumes large amounts of VOCs. Easy to grow, drought tolerant, disease resistant, and tolerant of city conditions, the Hollywood Juniper is a true Super-Tree. Hollywood Juniper is also often used as a large evergreen shrub. Winter hardy in zones 6–10.

Juniperus scopulorum 'Admiral' is another Super-Tree that is quite similar to 'Blue Heaven' but that grows slightly larger. 'Admiral,' despite the masculine name, is a pollen-free female and an excellent VOC remover. 'Admiral' is quite cold hardy but is also well adapted to growing in warm areas such as Los Angeles. Winter hardy in zones 3–10.

Juniperus scopulorum 'Blue Heaven' is a pyramidal-shaped evergreen tree, growing to about twenty feet tall. It is winter hardy, handsome, common in nurseries, and has beautiful bright blue-gray foliage. 'Blue Heaven,' a VOC consumer, female, and pollen free, is a fine evergreen Super-Tree. Winter hardy in zones 4–10.

Juniperus scopulorum 'Spearmint' is a narrow, upright-growing female Super-Tree that reaches a height of around twelve feet. 'Spearmint' is common in the trades and is well adapted to growing in mild-winter areas. 'Spearmint' would make an excellent substitute for the high-allergy, profuse pollen-producing, and often all too common Italian Cypress. Winter hardy in zones 4–10.

Juniperus squamata 'Meyeri' is commonly called the Meyer Juniper, the Fishback Juniper, or the Fishtail Juniper. Meyer Juniper matures as a broad, shrubby tree, often more than thirty feet tall. Meyer Juniper is a VOC remover and is pollen free. It is a common, widely used Super-Tree that is, as often as not, grown as a large shrub. Winter hardy in zones 4–10.

Juniperus virginiana 'Canaertii' is fairly common in the United States but is probably more common in Europe. These get to be large trees, reaching sixty feet or more where the soil is good and the rainfall abundant. 'Canaertii' is a female tree, making many blue berries among the bright, light green foliage. Cold hardy and widely adapted, 'Canaertii' is an excellent big Super-Tree and would make a fine substitute for pollen-producing redwoods or the larger cypress species. Winter hardy in zones 4–10.

Juniperus virginiana 'Pendula Chamberlaynii' is also called the Weeping Red Cedar. A large tree, it is widely adapted, a VOC consumer, and always female. There is a very similar tree, *Juniperus virginiana* 'Pendula Virdis,' which is also a fine Super-Tree. Be aware, though, that there is a ground cover clone sold under a similar name, *Juniperus virginiana* 'Pendula,' which is a male and has plenty of pollen. Winter hardy in zones 4–10.

Freeman Hybrid Maple 'Autumn Fantasy' *(Acer × Freemanii)* may also be sold as Hybrid Red Maple 'Autumn Fantasy.' This Super-Tree is a hybrid between a Red Maple and a Silver Maple. 'Autumn Fantasy' is a female tree, pollen free, and it is also an excellent net VOC remover. The original 'Autumn Fantasy' is a large female tree growing in central Illinois. A strong growing, hardy, robust Super-Tree, it is well known for its intense crimson fall color. Winter hardy in zones 4–10.

Red Maple 'Bowhall' *(Acer rubrum)* is another excellent female Super-Tree that has great fall color and exceptional air-cleaning abilities. 'Bowhall' grows very upright when young and eventually matures into a very symmetrical pyramidal form. Winter hardy in zones 4–9.

Red Maple 'Davey Red' *(Acer rubrum)* is another excellent Super-Tree with outstanding ability to remove pollen and VOCs. 'Davey Red' is a large female tree that has superior fall color and extra winter hardiness. It is sometimes also sold under as *Acer rubrum,* Red Maple, 'Davey.' Winter hardy in zones 3–9.

Red Maple 'Doric' *(Acer rubrum)* is a smaller Super-Tree but one that landscapers often find useful because of its narrow, columnar shape. Bright orange or red fall colors are an added attraction on this female tree that will clean air of both pollen and VOCs. Winter hardy in zones 3–9.

Red Maple 'October Glory' *(Acer rubrum)* is a large growing, widely adapted female Red Maple Super-Tree that is available at many nurseries. 'October Glory' is an excellent choice for cleaning the air of both pollen and VOCs. As an added plus, this tree has exceptional fall color. Winter hardy in zones 3–10.

Red Maple 'Red Sunset' *(Acer rubrum)* was introduced by Schmidt Nursery in Boring, Oregon, in 1966 and has since been a very popular maple. Its red-orange fall color is exceptional and long lasting. 'Red Sunset,' which is sometimes also sold as *Acer rubrum* 'Franksred,' is widely adapted to many different climates and soils. A large, healthy tree, it is another fine female Super-Tree with great ability to cleanse the air of pollen and VOCs. Winter hardy in zones 3–10.

Silver Maple 'Northline' *(Acer saccharinum 'Northline')* is a true Super-Tree in all respects. It is a large, deciduous female tree and removes much pollen from the air. It is extremely winter hardy even into zone 2 and is widely adaptable, growing well in many areas and in different soil types. Stronger branched than many other Silver Maples, 'Northline' is also especially good at removing huge amounts of harmful VOCs from the air. Winter hardy in zones 2–10.

Southern Red Maple 'San Felipe' *(Acer rubrum var. Drummondii 'San Felipe')* is a large, beautiful, female, deciduous tree that is better suited to warmer southern areas than are most Red Maples. 'San Felipe' has very large leaves and attractive, extra large, bright red seeds. This is one of the very best of any trees for cleaning maple pollen from the air and also for removing VOCs. For suitable southern areas, few trees would deserve to be called Super-Trees as much as 'San Felipe.' Winter hardy in zones 6–10.

All female, **fruiting mulberry trees (*Morus* species)** are true Super-Trees. These grow large, produce fruit for birds, produce no pollen, trap considerable amounts of pollen, dust, and other airborne particulates, and remove large amounts of carbon monoxide and ozone (VOCs). White mulberry, *Morus alba,* has fruit that is tasty but because of its light color is less attractive to birds (thus less messy). Winter hardy in zones 4–10.

Weeping Mulberry is almost always a pollen-free female clone, and its fruit, although purple, is rarely abundant.

Teeny-Tiny and Dangerous

In addition to VOCs, we are also faced with the problem of increasing amounts of generalized junk in our air. Very tiny airborne particles are often grouped together and called "particulates." Many, if not all, of these can aggravate allergies and asthma. The worst particulates come from these sources: dust from unpaved roads; smoke from wildfires, from prescribed burns, from agricultural residue burns; and smoke from wood-burning stoves and fireplaces. Also contributing to airborne-particulate levels are diesel exhaust, gasoline exhaust, industrial combustion, pollution from charbroilers and fryers, and wear from both brakes and tires. The wearing down of the millions of tires produces large amounts of airborne rubber particulates and contributes considerably to the growing incidence of dangerous latex allergies.

Anything we can do to limit the amount of particulates in our air is good and makes the air cleaner for us all.

VOC Control and Allergy-Free Gardening: Are They in Conflict?

It might well seem as though VOC control and allergy-free gardening do not mesh, especially since some plants with excellent OPALS rankings are also high VOC emitters. For example, a 'Theves' poplar, which is a pollen-free female poplar tree with excellent shape and growth characteristics, is nonetheless a VOC producer. How can it still deserve a great OPALS ranking then?

The answer is that it depends on where a tree like this is used. If you live in the country or in an area where the population is sparse and there is little or no smog problem, then there would only be limited NOx in the air.

In order for smog to be created, there must be a combination of sunlight, heat, VOCs, and NOx. Since NOx is mostly produced from engines, it is abundant in the city but not in the country.

Essentially this means that a high-VOC tree is only a smog tree when it is growing in the city. In someone's yard out in the country, it makes perfect sense to use female trees of any species. High-VOC trees that are pollen-free females, such as the above-mentioned 'Theves' Poplar; the weeping willow *(Salix babylonica);* or perhaps the pollen-free cultivar of Sour Gum, *Nyssa sylvatica* 'Miss Scarlet,' would still make excellent choices for an allergy-free landscape if you do not live in the city.

Conversely, if you do live in a city where smog is a concern, then by all means avoid planting new trees with high VOC ratings. Instead use those fine trees that combine the best of both, the pollen-free, VOC-removing Super-Trees.

CHAPTER 17

Random Facts, Odds and Ends with No Particular Place to Go

Oftentimes people who have allergies struggle to be in control, to feel good, to make sense out of their condition. Allergies are exceptionally individualistic; what affects one person may not affect another. All too often people without allergies are unsympathetic, and on TV those with allergies or asthma are often ridiculed or made the butt of jokes. If you have allergies, you need every bit of useful information you can get your hands on. Since avoidance is the key to success with allergies, having the right information is crucial. In this last chapter of *Safe Sex in the Garden* you'll find lots of allergy tidbits that may well be of use to you.

Shellac and the Cashew Family

At one time shellac was frequently used to coat wooden furniture. It is still occasionally used, mostly on imported materials. Shellac is a varnish regurgitated by tiny female scalelike insects, *Laccifer (Tachardia) lacca* (called "lac bugs"), feeding on trees that are in the huge and very allergenic Anacardiaceae family. This big group of plants is also called the Cashew family and includes landscape species like pepper trees and wild plants like poison ivy.

Shellac, which is often extremely allergenic, is usually imported from India. Shellac is generally only used on materials for inside the house, since it does not provide good protection against moisture. This may well be the reason people put coasters under glasses on tables. With modern polyurethane finishes, coasters really aren't needed.

Contact with shellacked furniture can cause serious allergic skin reactions, often from antique desks that were shellacked many years ago. The allergic response is usually a delayed reaction, hours or days after contact, making it difficult to track down.

Shellac for furniture can be replaced with either epoxy or polyurethane, which are certainly less allergenic. On numerous websites shellac is still sold and promoted, ironically often as the "nontoxic" product. Shellac is sometimes used in hair sprays (pump sprays or aerosol sprays with propan-butan or DME). Shellac may be used in hair-setting lotions and shampoos as well as in mascara, eyeliner, nail polish, and even lipstick.

Microencapsulation of shellac allows it to be used in fragrances and perfume oils. Shellac can occasionally be found in chewing gum, candies, cakes, eggs, or as a coating of citrus fruits and apples. Shellac is even used sometimes as a coating for pharmaceutical products, especially in slow-release tablets.

In the nutritional supplement industry (think vitamins), shellac is sometimes described as a "pharmaceutical food glaze." Some industries call shellac "lac resin." Other industries may call it "resinous glaze." Shellac may go by many different names.

Providing a glossy finish, shellac is used as a confectioner's glaze, which lengthens the shelf life of pan-coated candies such as chocolate-covered almonds. My advice is that everyone with allergies avoid shellac. Shellac is usually much more allergenic as a contact allergen, on the skin, but eating it really isn't a good idea either. Skin conditions caused by shellac are often very severe and hard to get rid of. Watch out for and avoid shellac!

People who are already allergic to poison oak, poison ivy, mangoes, or cashews are by far the most susceptible to shellac-caused dermatitis. All the members of this family can interreact with each other, and this is certainly worth noting.

I have a personal story, not about shellac but about its relatives, I want to tell you. A few years ago I'd been hiking and got lost. I ended up having to climb straight up several hundred feet of poison oak–covered rock. It was one of those situations where it was safer to go up than down, and I just plowed through it as best I could.

Although I scrubbed myself down afterward, I still broke out with a nasty case of poison oak rash all over my body. The doctors gave me prednisone, which eventually got the rash under control. One day when the rash was almost gone, except for a tiny bit left on my hands, I went for a long drive with my sister and brother-in-law. We were going from San Luis Obispo to San Diego, a drive of about three hundred miles. Not long into the drive, my sister broke out a huge bag of salted cashews and offered me some. I declined, saying that my poison oak was almost gone, and knowing what I did, I didn't want to push my luck. I drank a soda instead.

But my all too human nature being what it was, after about one hundred miles of driving, the salty cashews started to look pretty good. By the time we got to San Diego I'd done my share to help finish off the bag.

By late afternoon that day my hands started to itch pretty bad again, and by nightfall both hands were once again covered with poison oak blisters. I'll let you draw your own moral for that story!

Red Pepper Berries

The red berries or "peppers" (also called "peppercorns") from *Schinus* species pepper trees are often mixed with black or white peppers and sold as a festive-looking mix. Black or white pepper, *Piper nigrum,* which is the true pepper, is not even related to the pepper trees. Pepper trees are poison ivy relatives (another Anacardiaceae relation), and their fruits or "peppers" are not edible, and they are often highly allergenic. Allergic reactions, which may cause symptoms similar to hay fever, skin rash, or asthma, are usually time delayed, often for as long as several days after using this "pepper" mix. Don't use this mix yourself and warn others about it. This is a product that ought to be promptly taken off the market.

Cottonwood "Cotton" Is Flying—Bad Company

Some time ago I saw the question below posted on an Internet gardening forum and decided to answer it:

"Does anyone else here really suffer from allergies when the seeds of cottonwood are flying? I *know* it is not the cottonwood, but I am really curious as to what is pollinating at the same time" (Diana Pederson, Ingham County, Michigan, Zone 5, United States, author of *Landscaping with Bible Plants*).

This was a question I'd been asked many times before, and I knew my answer would be useful in *Safe Sex in the Garden*. So I saved it to share with you here. Please note that the author of this email is a garden writer herself and obviously more horticulturally savvy than most. Her question is a very good one.

Around here, in late spring, as the "cotton" (the seeds) of the female poplars (cottonwoods and aspens) and the willows is flying about, so is a good deal of pollen from different, unrelated species of trees. It is very common at this precise time that many people suffer from extreme bouts of hay fever, and often it is this "cotton" that gets the blame. Some city arborists refuse to plant female willows or poplars because of their firm (if mistaken) belief that this "cotton" is really some kind of pollen. But it isn't pollen; it is seed. It is *not* what is causing the allergies at that time.

By the time the seeds of the female willows and cottonwoods are flying, pollen from the males of these two species has already long since been released. This flying of cottony seed, however, coincides with the pollen release of many allergenic plants.

This is often the exact same time that the millions of urban "fruitless" male mulberry trees are shedding their prodigious and highly allergenic pollen. It is also the time that the olive trees are starting to release pollen. The cypress trees and shrubs are releasing very large amounts of pollen at this time too, as are the many male *Ailanthus* trees (Tree-of-Heaven). At or about that same time the walnut trees are releasing a large amount of pollen, as are many species of hickory, butternut, ginkgo, and pecan. Perhaps the most pervasive at this point are the oaks, many species of which are still at this time covered with staminate flowers and just loaded with pollen.

At the same time that the female willows and cottonwoods are releasing all that harmless fluff into the air, the birch trees have just finished shedding large amounts of pollen, much of which is still lying around on the ground. In southern areas the alders often bloom twice (as will many birch and junipers), and the second bloom of the alders sometimes will coincide precisely with the flying of the "cotton."

Moreover, when the cottony seeds of the willows and poplars start to float about, most of the male maples, male yews, male podocarpus, male pepper trees, male pistache, male junipers, male ash, and a large number of other landscape trees and shrubs have already released their own pollen. Unless this pollen was washed away by strong downpours of rain, much of it is still lying about and is still causing problems, weeks or sometimes even months after it was released.

To add to all of the above, at precisely this same time, the grasses start to release pollen. The ornamental landscape clump grasses all produce huge amounts of pollen at this time, as do most bluegrass and Bermuda lawns that have not been kept closely mowed.

By the time this cotton is in the air, many people with allergies are already starting to suffer from "systems overload." There is so much pollen being released and so much just released that it overwhelms the immune systems of many individuals. The innocent female cottonwoods are running with some bad company, and they're getting all the blame.

Aspirin Intolerance

About 5 to 6 percent of the general population are intolerant of aspirin, but among those with asthma as many as 20 percent may be aspirin sensitive. Reactions to aspirin intolerance may be itching, hay fever–like symptoms, or asthma. This is sometimes called "aspirin-induced asthma," or AIA.

Sulfites

Sulfites, a preservative, can be found in red or white wine, wine coolers, some beer, and especially on shrimp. Allergic reaction to sulfites can be immediate or delayed and severe, often with sudden itch, rash, breathing problems, red eyes, and/or shock. If you suspect this allergy, never eat anything you suspect may have shrimp in it until you have been assured that it does not. Be sure to ask and explain just how allergic to shrimp you are. This is a very dangerous allergy.

Many a wine lover has had to give up drinking wine when he or she keeps developing red, itchy rashes from the sulfites in the wine. Rash from sulfites in wine usually shows up first on the neck, shoulders, or back.

Tourette's Syndrome

There appears to be a strong connection to Tourette's Syndrome (TS) and allergies. In one family that had seven members with TS, all seven of them also had pollen allergies. People with TS should be especially careful to avoid well-known allergens such as pollen and mold.

More on Rubber (Latex) Allergies

There appears to be widespread confusion between the terms "rubber" allergy and "latex" allergy. Actually they are usually the exact same thing. Most rubber comes from the latex sap of the tropical tree *Hevea brasiliensis*, a *Euphorbia* family member. Rubber is used in making tires, hoses, foam rubber, latex or rubber gloves, pencil erasers, rubber balls, and many other common products. Latex is potentially a serious allergen for a large and growing number of people.

Rubber allergy has become much more common since the advent of AIDS and the related wearing of rubber gloves. This dangerous allergy is growing rapidly among medical workers, police, firefighters, and people who have had multiple surgical operations. Very serious reactions have occurred from contact with surgical tubing and other latex surgical equipment. Dental patients whose mouths were covered with rubber dams have experienced reactions of dangerous facial swelling.

Not So Safe Sex?

A growing number of men, and some women also, have been experiencing painful allergic reaction after using latex condoms. In France they have developed a deproteinized latex condom that has proved to be safe in tests.

Rubber allergies are potentially deadly. Cross-species-reactive rubber allergy from pollen or sap of other *Euphorbia* family members is quite possible. People with allergy to rubber should avoid having any of these plants as houseplants, shrubs, trees, or vines.

The Euphorbiaceae (Spurge group) is a very large and popular horticultural family of plants with over 280 different genera and more than 7,000 species. The Spurge family includes (but is not limited to) plants in the generas (plural of genus) *Acalypha*, *Bischofia*, *Cnidoscolus*, *Croton*, *Elaephorbia*, *Euphorbia*, *Garcia*, *Hevea*, *Hura*, *Jatropha*, *Manihot*, *Monadenium*, *Ricinus*, *Sapium*, and *Tetracoccus*. Many of these plants are separate sexed (dioecious), and the males, since they produce pollen, present additional health hazards.

Recently some children playing in fast-food ball pits have suffered allergic anaphylactic shock. The balls themselves were plastic, but they were latex-contaminated because the floors of the pits were covered with thick rubber foam linings.

I recently saw a lady with rubber allergy who suddenly became terribly sick while she was sitting in the waiting room of a tire store, waiting for her car's tires to be changed. There were many tires in the waiting room, and the entire immediate area would no doubt have a considerable amount of airborne rubber particles in it from the changing of all those tires. If you have a rubber allergy, get a friend to take your car to the tire store for you. One of the most common allergic reactions to rubber is swelling, often facial swelling. Other common reactions are itching and a feeling that it is hard to breathe (which may be if your airways are also swelling, choking off your air supply).

Also, if you even suspect you may be allergic to rubber, do not ever blow up any balloons.

Other Plant Species Latex Concerns

People with rubber allergy may be at increased risk of becoming sensitive to latex sap from species of plants that are unrelated to the *Euphorbias*. Latex sap from *Ficus* trees would be just one example of this. For those with rubber allergies, it is a good idea to avoid contact with any milky, white, "latex-looking" plant sap. Anyone who suspects that they may be allergic to rubber would be wise to carefully read chapter 9 on plants that may cause skin rashes.

Weight Gain and Weight Loss

There is considerable evidence that allergies can cause some people to gain weight and others to lose weight. Usually, it seems, that those who'd like to gain weight, lose, and those who'd like to lose, gain. This is an area certainly worth exploring, but at the present time, while recognized, it is not generally well understood.

Allergies are well known to cause many people to lose their sense of smell, and some also lose their sense of taste. This situation could cause some folks to lose interest in eating.

At the same time, the flip side can also be at work with weight gain. Allergies also can make any attempt at exercise seem worthless, and this inactivity itself could lead to weight gain.

Allergies can also make some people retain a considerable amount of water in their body, most often in their face, hands, and feet. Some allergy medicines also cause fluid retention.

Air-Conditioning and Heater Ducts

Ever looked inside your air-conditioning and heating vents? Over time, air ducts can easily become traps for pollen, dirt, dust, and other contaminants like mildew, mold, fungus, animal dander, dust mites, and bacteria. These pollutants can recirculate in the air when you turn on the air-conditioning or heating.

Change air-conditioning filters often and regularly. Hire professionals who specialize in this to clean heater and air-conditioning ducts.

Sometimes air-conditioning tubes in automobiles will also be moldy and will need cleaning. There are some very good, easy to use products for this. Check the "Useful Websites" section of this book (page 202).

Swamp coolers can also grow mold, so these too need to be cleaned several times a season. In some cases it may pay to run a solution of bleach and water through the swamp cooler for a few minutes to kill molds. Make sure the house is well ventilated when you do this!

Some experts recommend that anyone with allergies avoid staying in hotel or motel rooms that are cooled with swamp coolers. These rooms are often filled with mold spores.

Air Filter Machines for the House

Some home air filter machines are just too noisy, and you'll soon tire of the noise. The best units are powerful, quiet, and have very fine, replaceable HEPA filters. (HEPA stands for highly-efficiency particulate air; HEPA filters will trap all pollen and most mold spores.) Avoid the fanless "ionic" type of air filters that supposedly attract air particles by osmosis. Some of these ionic cleaners give off a bad smell, and many people feel that none of them cleans air all that well. Some ionic cleaners have also been implicated as giving off ozone, which is itself an allergen.

With clean air machines you often get what you pay for, and the best units are not cheap. See the "Useful Websites" section (page 202) for places to shop for air cleaners.

Allergic to Sunlight

There are a number of diseases that are caused or triggered by exposure to bright sunlight. The most common of these is PMLE, which stands for polymorphic light eruption. This is often confused with another sunlight-caused response called "prickly heat."

Typical symptoms of PMLE are small red itchy eruptions on the skin.

Also occurring more frequently is lupus, which also often results in supersensitivity to heat and bright sunlight.

It is not well understood what initially causes any of these illnesses, but people who have them frequently also suffer from pollen allergies. Anyone with PMLE or lupus would be wise to avoid excessive pollen levels whenever possible. There are also some good lightweight, high-tech clothes now available that protect the skin and make it possible for these people to get outside more, even on sunny days. See the "Useful Websites" section (page 202) for these clothes.

Female Lawns

There are now a number of female, pollen-free types of lawn grass sod available. These are clonal selections of Buffalo Grass, *Buchloe dactyloides,* a native grass that grew where the buffalo used to roam. These are warm-season grasses that will go completely dormant in the winter months, but they are still very useful for numerous reasons. Female selections of Buffalo Grass need very little, if any, mowing. They grow and stay quite short, and some are an attractive green-blue color. These selections also are exceptionally drought tolerant and once established need far less irrigation than most other lawns. They are also useful for covering no-mow slopes.

These female selections must be purchased as either sod or plugs. If not available in your area yet, these clonal female grasses can be bought through mail order. If grown from seed, both male and female plants will be present, and the pollen of the males is potent. Female lawns are the way of the future, and for anyone concerned with grass pollen, they are well worth considering. See the "Useful Websites" section (page 202) for more information.

Fumes from Microwave Popcorn

Recently it was discovered that many people who worked where microwave popcorn was produced were suffering with serious lung conditions from the fumes. While this is not an allergic response per se, anything that damages the lungs makes people more susceptible to allergies. With this in mind, it would be a very sensible thing for us to make sure that if and when we microwave popcorn ourselves, we keep windows wide open and exhaust fans on.

Fumes from Burned Teflon Pans

Fumes produced when Teflon pans are burned can cause serious damage to the lungs. Sometimes this damage can be permanent. If you use Teflon pans (and who doesn't?), take extra care not to let them sit on the stove too long. Also, if you find that you or a loved one is in the habit of having this happen, a switch to cast-iron pans would be a good idea. Again, while this is not directly allergy-related, impaired lungs will always have an extra bad effect on those with asthma or allergies.

Since we're talking about pots and pans here, it is wise to remember that aluminum can escape during cooking and that it is a very toxic chemical. People with allergies need to take extra care with all toxic elements, which can leave them ever-more susceptible to allergens. Again, a switch from aluminum pans to cast-iron pots and pans is worth considering.

Sludge

This product, which is composted waste from sewage treatment facilities, is sold as a soil amendment. It does have good qualities, but it also contains dangerous heavy metals. These heavy metals can be taken up by our plants and can end up in our fruit and vegetables. Don't use sludge around your fruit trees or in your vegetable gardens. Actually, better not to use it at all.

Mushroom Compost

In many areas it is possible to buy the used soil from mushroom growers, which is sold as mushroom compost. People with allergies should be aware that this material is loaded with fungus spores and just spreading it can trigger an allergic attack. Use only with care.

Edible Flowers and Herbal Tea

There are a great many flowers that are eaten fresh in salads, or often dried and used as ingredients in herbal teas. Keep in mind that many of these have fully developed male stamens and that the pollen can cause allergies. With some flowers, such as *Feijoa sellowiana*, pineapple guava, only the sweet fleshy sepals are used, and these contain no pollen. Sudden, severe attacks of asthma, however, have been brought on by drinking, in particular, chamomile tea. But any herbal tea containing flowers should be used with caution by those with allergies. If an itchy throat or any such sign of allergy is detected after drinking any of these herbal teas, take that as a warning and avoid them in the future.

Old Straw Mulch

Old hay makes very good mulch in the vegetable garden, but it should be used with caution. Often hay that was baled too moist will be moldy and unfit to use for fodder. This same hay may be given away as mulch, but the spores released from it while being spread can cause a permanent condition known as "farmers' lung."

Hay that was baled late will be full of flowers and pollen. Straw, left over from grain crops, will also be full of pollen.

The very best hay for mulch is the same as the very best hay for fodder. It is hay that was cut early, prebloom cut hay. This hay will have much less pollen, will be free of mold, it will have few weed seeds, and it also adds the most nutrient value for the soil.

Fast Relief

Many people who are suffering from allergies find that breathing steamed air makes them feel better. If hay fever or asthma is keeping you awake at night, using a warm humidifier often helps. Put the humidifier in a small bathroom and turn it up as warm and moist as possible. These units are inexpensive and easy to use. Sit in the bathroom and just breathe in the moist, warm air, and often you'll get some fast relief. Allergies and asthma both can cause shortness of breath, and this in turn causes more rapid breathing. The extra effort seems to dry out the mouth and bronchial tubes; thus extra humidity makes it easier to breathe.

There is a down side to this though. Your bathroom can get moldy from all the extra moisture. Be sure to air it out very well in between sessions with the humidifier.

When you're outside working in the garden on a day with plenty of pollen about, remember that pollen easily sticks to clothing and hair. As soon as you come inside, try this great tip passed on to me by the garden writer Carol Deppe. Once in the house, boil some water and breathe in some of the steam. Then quickly wash your face and hands, brush your hair, and change your shirt. Often this makes a world of difference.

Taking Advantage of a Lake or the Ocean—or Not

Many people have found that when their allergies are at their worst, they feel better just sitting at the edge of a large lake or right next to the ocean. Since there are no trees, shrubs, or grasses growing on the water, the air coming across it is very clean and fresh. Sitting next to a large body of water like this can clean out your lungs and leave you feeling much better. For some people, living near the ocean is by far the best way to feel good.

RED TIDES

An exception to the above advice exists when there are red tides. Red tides can be fairly common along the coast in some areas in late summer and fall. These are especially common along the Gulf of Mexico. The red tides are caused by a huge bloom of algae, and in the process billions of spores are released into the air. People fishing, working, or just walking along the shore during a red tide can quickly fall ill. Symptoms usually include coughing, irritated throat, eyes, nose, and other flu-like symptoms. Everyone, but especially those with allergies, should avoid the shoreline if there is a red tide in process.

Christmas Trees

Recently some people have been selling Leylandii Cypress trees as allergy-free Christmas trees. The claim is that they are pollen free. I would recommend a Norfolk Island Pine over a Leylandii Cypress tree for an allergy-free Christmas tree. Leylandii Cypress are *not* pollen-free trees, although their pollen is usually sterile. Sterile pollen though is by no means necessarily nonallergenic. In some species sterile pollen is indeed less allergenic, but in other species it is as allergenic as is viable pollen. Also, Leylandii Cypress is a cypress hybrid, and Cypress is a very highly allergenic family, one of the worst.

Norfolk Island Pines (*Araucaria excelsior*) are not true pines, and they lack most of the smell associated with evergreen conifers. They will not produce any pollen until they are very large trees, and never as a potted, living Christmas tree.

I would suggest that anyone using any real tree as a Christmas tree spray it thoroughly with Wiltpruff, which is a water-soluble waxy substance. Wiltpruff is used to hold in moisture, so it will keep the trees from drying out so quickly. Sprayed on right, it will also lock in most of the available pollen, mold spores, and even a considerable amount of the smell.

Woodworking and Sawdust

Many gardeners also like to do some woodworking. Please keep the following in mind: there are many illnesses and allergies associated with contact with sawdust. Sawdust from some trees is much worse than others (in general hardwoods are more dangerous than softwoods), but all wood dust is suspect. Especially dangerous is the wood dust from fine sanding, since it is so small and can be inhaled deep into the lung.

Some problems commonly associated with prolonged contact to sawdust and other types of wood dusts are asthma, allergic skin rashes, irritation and inflammation of the eyes, and nasal cancers. Use a facemask when sanding wood and always treat sawdust with caution.

A few types of lumber to watch out for in particular are:

Acacia – Sawdust is a potential carcinogen.

Black Locust – Sawdust can irritate skin and nauseates some people.

Maple – Sawdust can cause numerous allergic responses.

Oak – Sawdust is a carcinogen and can cause asthma.

Olivewood – Sawdust can irritate skin, eyes, and nose.

Western Red Cedar – Sawdust may cause asthma or other allergic reactions.

Yew wood – Sawdust is toxic.

More on Particulates

Anyone with allergies ought to take extra care when using any material that is fine grained and/or possibly dusty. Make a concerted effort not to expose yourself to breathing in facial powders, talcum powder, dust from flour or nondairy creamers, or dust from vermiculite or perlite. When using dry manure or any kind of potting soil, peat moss, or soil amendments in the garden, be sure not to inhale any dust from them. These may be full of mold spores, and the minute pieces of the material (the particulates) themselves may trigger allergies.

Pollen and Pregnant Women

A study from Sweden (delivered at the European Respiratory Society in Stockholm on September 16, 2002) found that babies are more likely to suffer from asthma if their mothers were exposed to pollen during the last three months of pregnancy. Swedish epidemiologist Bertil Forsberg and colleagues studied 111,702 babies conceived between 1988 and 1995 in the Stockholm area. Their report states, "It is clear that maternal pollen exposure in the last 12 weeks of pregnancy plays a major role [in the development of asthma in babies]."[1]

So, what does this mean for us? It is yet another piece of the big puzzle. It reinforces my findings that excessive pollen is a major biopollutant and a serious health hazard. And the most obvious lesson here is that expectant women need to take special care to avoid large amounts of pollen toward the end of their pregnancies.

INTRODUCTION

1. Brunekreef, Bert, Gerard Hoek, Paul Fischer, and Frits Spieksma. 2000. "Relation between airborne pollen concentrations and daily cardiovascular and respiratory-disease mortality." *The Lancet* 355:9214.

CHAPTER 1

1. Brunekreef, Bert, Gerard Hoek, Paul Fischer, and Frits Spieksma. 2000. "Relation between airborne pollen concentrations and daily cardiovascular and respiratory-disease mortality." *The Lancet* 355: 9214.

CHAPTER 14

1. Cimons, Marlene. March 21, 2001. "CDC to Detial Blood Contaminants." *The Los Angeles Times*, A5

CHAPTER 15

1. LaDeau, Shannon L. and J. S. Clark. April 6, 2001. "Rising CO_2 levels and the fecundity of forest trees." *Science* 292:95–98.

2. Global warming's high carbon dioxide levels may exacerbate ragweed allergies. August 15, 2000. USDA (Press) Release No. 0278.00.

3. Tuchman, Nancy C., Robert G. Wetzel, Steven T. Rier, Kirk A. Wahtera, and James A. Teeri. 2002. "Elevated atmospheric

CO_2 lowers leaf litter nutritional quality for stream ecosystem food webs." *Global Change Biology* 8(2):163–170.

CHAPTER 17

1. Forsberg, Bertil, Mara Slavkovic-Jovanovic, Sheelagh Fleming, Seif Shaheen, Mohammad Shamssain, and Stephen W. Turner. September 16, 2002. "Babies are three times as likely to suffer from asthma in their first year if their mothers were exposed to pollen in the last trimester of pregnancy." European Respiratory Society 12th Annual Congress Press Release.

RECOMMENDED READING

This list of references is in no way complete, but included are a few of the books and articles that I found especially useful in the writing of *Safe Sex in the Garden* and *Allergy-Free Gardening*. Some are chiefly about allergies, and others are specifically about horticulture.

Bailey, Liberty Hyde, and Ethel Zoe Bailey, eds. *Hortus Third: A Concise Dictionary of Plants Cultivated in the United States and Canada.* New York: Collier Macmillan Publishers, 1976. A book I use daily.

Brenzel, Kathleen Norris, ed. *Sunset Western Garden Book.* Menlo Park, Calif.: Lane Publishing Company, 2001. For the western United States, this is still one of the most useful general gardening books. The newest edition is a beautiful book.

Cairns, Thomas, ed. *Modern Roses XI: The World Encyclopedia of Roses.* San Diego, Calif.: Academic Press, 2000. For serious rose lovers, this is *the* book.

Deppe, Carole. *Breed Your Own Vegetable Varieties: The Gardener's and Farmer's Guide to Plant Breeding and Seed Saving.* White River Junction, Vt.: Chelsea Green Publishing Company, 2000. An excellent book for those wishing to try their own hand at plant breeding.

Dirr, Michael A. *Dirr's Hardy Trees and Shrubs: An Illustrated Encyclopedia.* Portland, Ore.: Timber Press, 1997. A well-written, useful reference book, but plugs use of male clones.

Flint, Harrison L. *Landscape Plants for Eastern North America.* New York: John Wiley & Sons, 1983. An older book but still a very good one.

Hiller, John, and Allen Coombes, eds. *The Hiller Manual of Trees and Shrubs*. Devon, England: David & Charles Publishers, 2002. One of the best guides for locating hard to find cultivars.

Jacobson, Arthur Lee. *North American Landscape Trees*. Berkeley, Calif.: Ten Speed Press, 1996. One of the very best books on hardy landscape trees. Jacobson understands sex systems in trees and always includes this information. Excellent attention to detail.

Jelks, M.D., Mary. *Allergy Plants*. Tampa, Fla.: World Wide Publications, 1997. All of Dr. Jelks's material is interesting and useful, and her photos are excellent.

Jury, S.L., Cutler Reynolds, and F. J. Evans. *The Euphorbiales: The Chemistry, Taxonomy and Economic Botany*. London, England: The Linnean Society of London, The Whitefriars Press, 1987. The book on the potent *Euphorbias*.

Lewis, Walter H., and Memory P. F. Elvin-Lewis. *Medical Botany: Plants Affecting Man's Health*. New York: John Wiley and Sons Publishers, 1977. Written by a dynamic botanist and microbiologist husband-wife team. On the subject of medical botany, this is *the* book.

——, Prathibha Vinay, and Vincent E. Zenger. *Airborne and Allergenic Pollen of North America*. Baltimore, Md.: The John Hopkins University Press, 1983. From a purely scientific point of view, I consider this the best book ever written on the connections between plants and pollen allergy.

McMinn, Howard E., and Evelyn Maino. *Pacific Coast Trees*. Berkeley: University of California Press, 1981. A fine, easy-to-use book for identifying West Coast trees.

Mortensen, Ernest, and Ervin Bullard. *Handbook of Tropical and Sub-Tropical Horticulture*. Washington D.C.: United States Department of Agriculture, Government Printing Office, 1964. Very useful book on tropicals.

Ogren, Thomas Leo. *Allergy-Free Gardening.* Berkeley, Calif.: Ten Speed Press, 2000.

Peattie, Donald Culross. *A Natural History of Trees.* 2 vols. Boston, Mass.: Houghton Mifflin Company, 1991. Originally published in 1948. If you love trees and fabulous nature writing, do yourself a favor and read these. Exceptionally well written, researched, and totally interesting.

Rapp, M.D., Doris. *Is This Your Child?* New York: William Morrow and Company, 1991. Doris Rapp is a true pioneer in allergy study.

Sargent, Charles Sprague. *Manual of the Trees of North America.* New York: Dover Publications, Inc., 1965. One of the very best tree books around.

Snyder, Leon C. *Gardening in the Upper Midwest.* Minneapolis: University of Minnesota Press, 1978. Fine book for zones 3–5 gardening.

Taylor, Norman. *Taylor's Encyclopedia of Gardening.* Cambridge, Mass.: Houghton Mifflin Co., 1948. This is an old but wonderful book. One of my all-time favorites, this is a very useful general gardening book. If you can find a copy, buy it!

Van Gelderen, D. M., P. C. de Jong, and H. J. Oterdoom. *Maples of the World.* Portland, Ore.: Timber Press, 1994. The very best book I've ever read on maples.

Wodehouse, R. P. *Pollen Grains.* New York: McGraw-Hill Book Company, 1935. Wodehouse was one of the first and one of the best pollen-allergy researchers. *Pollen Grains* is a classic in allergy literature.

www.aanma.org – Website of Mother of Asthmatics. An impressive organization.

www.achooallergy.com/ – Is another good source for anti-allergy products, filters, cleaners, etc.

www.allegra.com/starting_low_allergen_garden.jsp – A pharmaceutical site that has extensive material on allergy-free gardening.

www.allergicchild.com/images/pollen_allergies.htm – Great site for parents with allergic children.

http://allergies.about.com/library/weekly/aa030501a.htm – About.com's Judy Tidwell does a great job of hosting this interactive allergy website.

www.allergybuyersclub.com/healthy_home.shtml – Here is a great source for high-quality indoor air cleaners, information, and advice.

www.allergyfree-gardening.com – This is my own website, and you can contact me, Tom Ogren, through this site.

www.allergypreventioncenter.com/index.html – Good site for allergy information and sharing of ideas.

www.backyardgardener.com – Another fun gardening site.

www.buildinggreen.com/index.html – An important website, from the editors of the ahead of its time publication *Environmental Building News.*

www.canadiangardening.com – Good site for Canadian gardeners.

www.cheshire.gov.uk/rhs2002/links.htm – Terrific garden site with many links. A UK site but with gardening links from all over the world.

www.consciouschoice.com – Interesting, cutting edge, health and social issues website.

www.earthisland.org – A take no prisoners green site, very interesting material here.

www.epa.gov/iaq/pubs/airclean.html – Government site on air filtering systems.

www.gardenclub.org – Site of the wonderful state garden clubs.

www.gardenforever.com/pages/artallergy.htm – Garden Forever is a fun and useful gardening link.

www.gardenguides.com – A wonderful resource for gardeners.

www.gardenofgood.com – Another good one.

http://go4green.sask.com/msu/msu002.html – Garden site edited by the terrific Ms. Understanding.

www.icangarden.com – One of my favorite gardening sites.

www.innerself.com/Environmental/allergy_epidemic.htm – *InnerSelf Magazine*'s interesting website.

www.lungusa.org/breatheasyoffice/landscape.html – Contains a description of their ground-breaking allergy-free landscape. No male trees here!

www.lungusa.org/virginia/press_ogren0202.html – Site of the American Lung Association of Virginia. This headquarters has the first ALA low-pollen landscape in the country.

www.nadca.com – Website of the National Air Duct Cleaners Association.

www.pioneerthinking.com/main.html – Interesting site for mind-body-health information.

www.simpleplanet.homestead.com – A wonderful website, back to the land material.

www.stepintothegarden.com/links/gardening.html – Big list of good gardening links.

www.suite101.com/links.cfm/allergies – Tons of good information and articles on allergy here.

www.sunprecautions.com – A good source for sun protection clothes for people with lupus.

www.tenspeedpress.com – Website of my favorite publisher.

www.thelaboroflove.com/websearch/links/Child/Health/Allergies/ – Good site for pregnant allergy sufferers.

www.treelink.org – Urban forestry site.

www.urban-forestry.com/citytrees/v36n4a15.html – Urban forest site, City Trees, lots of useful information here.

www.weather.com/activities/health/allergies/ – Weather Channel has some interesting material on allergies and lots of pollen counts.

ABOUT THE AUTHOR

Thomas Leo Ogren has a master's degree in agriculture, with an emphasis on plant flowering systems and their relationship to allergy. He is a horticulturist and allergy researcher as well as a former nursery owner and has taught landscape gardening for twenty years. He is a consultant for the American Lung Association, the USDA, and Allegra. He is the author of *Allergy-Free Gardening*, and *Safe Sex in the Garden* is his fourth book. His work on allergies has been seen on TV shows, including the Canadian Discovery Channel. He writes for *New Scientist, Grandiflora, Alernative Medicine, Landscape Architecture,* and many other publications. Tom lives with his family in San Luis Obispo, California.

His email address is tloallergyfree@earthlink.net.